RADICAL
LOVING
CARE

"[Chapman] has written a book that should be in the hands of every healthcare executive who truly believes in the core mission of taking care of others . . . Anyone who leads a healthcare organization of any kind should read this book."

— **Chuck Lauer**, *publisher of* Modern Healthcare *magazine*

"Splendid, poetic, and eminently practical. I shall be recommending it highly to all the health care organizations I visit. Erie Chapman is a beacon of light in American Health care. With *Radical Loving Care* as a practical guide, no leader has the excuse now not to take their hospital system in a more imaginative and healing direction. A profoundly moving exploration combined with a detailed roadmap to something better, this book is a sure companion on the way to something much, much better: a hospital we might actually look forward to entering during the great transitions of life and death."

— **David Whyte**, *best-selling author of* The Heart Aroused *and* Crossing the Unknown Sea

"Erie Chapman has identified where we all want to be and he has given us a roadmap to get there. The Rings of Care concept alone is worth the read."

— **Bonnie Phipps**, *CEO,* Saint Joseph's Health System, Atlanta

"Erie Chapman has clearly articulated the true role of health care leadership…to promote a culture of Radical loving care."

— **Jim Nathan**, *President and CEO,* Lee Memorial Health System, Fort Myers, Florida

"Radical Loving Care offers a concept of humanism that sets a new standard."

— **Dr. Thomas W. Chapman**, *President and CEO,* The HSC Foundation, Washington, D.C.

"*Radical Loving Care* takes patient-centered care to a new level. This is a must read for not only caregivers but health care executives as well."
— ***Gail Warden***, *President Emeritus,*
Henry Ford Health System, Detroit

"Mr. Chapman delivers a clarion call to action by reminding all of us in healthcare that we must nurture the soul as well as treat the body if we are to be true healers. He not only provides a concise blueprint for how hospitals can achieve 'loving care,' but he also demonstrates how it makes good business sense to do so."
— ***Ed Eckenoff***, *President and CEO,*
National Rehabilitation Hospital Network

"Erie Chapman has described the special qualities that separate the good from the great in people and in organizations. What a different place the world would be if we could all live out his healing model."
— ***Michael Means***, *President and CEO,*
Health First, Melbourne, Florida

"Erie Chapman's book brings a powerful and important message to everyone involved in patient care. This is a passionate guidebook written by a man who has already demonstrated extraordinary leadership in healthcare."
— ***Martha H. Marsh***, *President and CEO,*
Stanford Hospitals and Clinics,
Palo Alto, California

"This book offers an oasis: the vision of a higher and more meaningful common ground. If we could establish the true healing health system within our communities, I suspect many of the 'business' problems in healthcare might suddenly have easier solutions."
— ***Robert Pallari***, *President and CEO,*
Legacy Health System,
Portland, Oregon

RADICAL
LOVING
CARE

Building the Healing Hospital in America

ERIE CHAPMAN

Printed in the United States of America

07 08 09 10 11 10 9 8

Library of Congress Control Number: 2003115640

ISBN 978-0-9747366-0-0

Eighth Printing - 2007

Cover and page design: Bill Kersey and Erie Chapman

Cover Painting: Highmore, Joseph *The Good Samaritan*, 1744. Tate Gallery, London, Great Britain. Photo credit: Tate Gallery, London

Back cover photo: Tia Ann Chapman, 2003

Printed at Vaughan Printing, Nashville

Published by:
Baptist Healing Hospital Trust
1919 Charlotte Avenue, Suite 320
Nashville, Tennessee 37203
(615) 284-8271
www.healinghospital.org
www.eriechapman.com

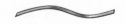

Other works by Erie Chapman

Books:
Life is Choices, Choose Well (CHI Press, 1995)

Films:
Acts of Caring — Produced and Directed by Erie Chapman (1993)

Sacred Work — (Baptist Healing Hospital Trust, 2001) — Produced and Directed by Erie Chapman, Editor, Van Grafton, Videography, Van Grafton and Andrew Haege

The Servant's Heart — the lives of four caregivers (Baptist Healing Hospital Trust, 2003) — Produced and Directed by Erie Chapman, Editor, Van Grafton, Director of Videography, Van Grafton

Music compositions:
Blessed Baby...and Other Sacred Music of Healing (Baptist Healing Hospital Trust, 2001)

Angel Hour — *Music of Healing from the film A Servant's Heart* (Baptist Healing Hospital Trust, 2003)

All of the above are available through:
www.healinghospital.com

Or through:
The Baptist Healing Hospital Trust
Nashville, Tennessee

Dedication

This work is dedicated to America's frontline caregivers,

those people who quietly and lovingly commit their lives to helping

the sick, the injured, and those laboring to bring new life into this world.

It is also dedicated to my tiny grandson, who will one day carry

forward the Golden Thread in his own loving hands.

Always act out of love,
not fear

The Healing Hospital™ Trinity

The caring culture of the Healing Hospital results from the conscious culti-vation of three themes: The GOLDEN THREAD OF HEALING *that is the <u>faith</u> legacy of our ancestors and the source of our calling as caregivers; the* SACRED WORK *that rises from our <u>hope</u> for meaningful experience as caregivers; and the* SERVANT'S HEART *that is grounded in a <u>love</u> that must go beyond ourselves. This trinity is the underpinning of the* **Healing Hospital**.

Other Loving Care Organizations

Although much of the content of this book references hospital examples, the model of The Healing Hospital should be easily adaptable to any organization focused on loving care. In particular, hospices, ambulatory clinics, mental health facilities, homeless shelters — any organization that seeks to serve, can benefit from the concepts and methods described in Radical Loving Care. *Examples of charitable organizations that are already putting the Healing Hospital model in place are Alive Hospice, under the direction of Jan Jones; the Siloam Clinic, under the leadership of Nancy West; and Interfaith Dental Clinic, under the guidance of Dr. Rhonda Switzer. We applaud these organi-zations for their enlightened thinking.*

Contents

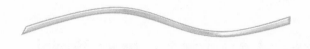

PART ONE
Love and the Higher Standard of the Healing Hospital

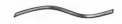

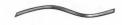

INTRODUCTORY NOTE

The ideas that make up this book have been taking shape for nearly the last three decades. Ever since I first entered a hospital as an inexperienced young executive in 1975, I have been fascinated by the way in which these complex organizations operate. I was struck first and foremost by how different a hospital seems when you look at it from within the operation contrasted with how it appears as a patient.

Before entering hospital leadership, I spent seven years as a trial attorney, the last three of them as a federal prosecuting attorney. On my second day on the job at Riverside Hospital in Toledo, a Code Blue was called over the P.A. system, signaling a patient with a heart attack. As an attorney, I was accustomed to responding to my client's emergencies. I knew little about hospitals, but it sounded like someone in the place I worked needed help. I jumped up from my chair and raced down the hallway toward the site of the Code. Halfway there, I slowed my pace and came to a stop. What was I going to do when I reached the heart attack victim? Draft a will? File a lawsuit?

Obviously, I wasn't trained to do anything that would be helpful to the patient. As I turned and walked back toward my office, I began to ask myself a question I've repeated many times since. What is the most important thing an executive does in leading a hospital? One thing I can say for sure. When a patient is admitted to the hospital, he or she never asks, "Hey, do they have enough executives here?" The patient wants medical help from a trained professional, not executive assistance from a guy like me in a suit.

Across the next twenty-seven years, during which I had the privilege of leading three large health systems in three parts of the country, I became clear on the answer to that question. Obviously, our hospitals' CEOs don't take care of patients. So, what *do* they do? The single most important thing a hospital CEO does is to take care of the people who take care of people — to serve the servers. It is when CEOs focus on this goal that hospitals excel.

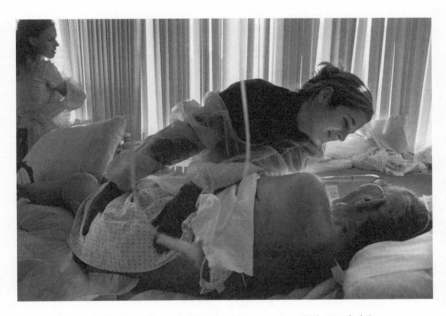

Photo — by Tia Ann Chapman, 2002, used by permission of *The Hartford Courant*

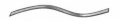

PART ONE

Love and
The Higher Standard
Of the Healing
Hospital

The Conceptual Foundations of Radical Loving Care

To love means to open ourselves to the negative as well as the positive — to grief, sorrow, and disappointment as well as to joy, fulfillment, and an intensity of consciousness we did not know was possible before.

— Dr. Rollo May

The hour is striking so close above me,
so clear and sharp,
that all my senses ring with it.
I feel it now: there's a power in me
to grasp and give shape to my world.
I know that nothing has ever been real
without my beholding it.
All becoming has needed me.
My looking ripens things
and they come toward me, to meet and be met.

— Rainer Maria Rilke

Chapter 1

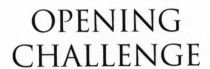

OPENING
CHALLENGE

Stories form the basis of vision.
— Professor Douglas Meeks, Vanderbilt Divinity School

THE HOUSEKEEPER AND THE OLD MAN

A veteran housekeeper swings her mop rhythmically along the linoleum-coated 7th-floor hallway of a large urban hospital. From a nearby room the cry of an old man who is confused by age and illness carves a ragged hole in the hallway air. He is begging for his absent daughter.

Calls of anguish and confusion come frequently from hospital rooms across America, but they are often ignored. The staff members are busy with other things.

After a little while, as the man continues to cry out, the housekeeper does something that is very unusual in the contemporary American hospital. Instead of ignoring the call or waiting for a nurse to respond, she puts down her mop, walks into the old man's room, and gently takes his hand in hers. The old man calms down immediately and soon goes off to sleep. The housekeeper returns to mopping the floor.

The housekeeper has quietly created what we call in a Healing Hospital a Sacred Encounter: Need has been heard and has been answered with love. For a few moments, she and the confused, sick old man have entered love's endless and immortal stream. In these moments the housekeeper has broken through the traditional bonds of her work, freed herself from the fear of being punished by a supervisor for stepping outside her job description, and responded to a human cry for help. The old man's call for love was answered — not by a drug or a patient restraint, but by the soothing touch of a loving hand.

A Healing Hospital is about loving service to others. It is about recognizing something that has increasingly been forgotten in a flood of the complex technology and magic-bullet drugs that now dominate America's hospitals. It is about the compassion and skill that must accompany the use of new technology and pharmaceuticals. And it is about the kind of leadership needed to support the underappreciated caregivers who staff America's hospitals.

The great unfinished business of healthcare is not curing but healing. Unfortunately, most of America's healthcare leaders are living a lie. They are promising loving care to the public in mission statements and then making no meaningful effort to ensure that care is actually practiced.

A Healing Hospital is not built with bricks and mortar. It is built with people who have Servant's Hearts, or a passion to serve, and who know that the fundamental relationship between caregiver and patient can be understood as a Sacred Encounter. It can be created in any healthcare setting where leaders and staff join together in a new commitment to what we call Radical Loving Care — creating a continuous chain of caring light around each and every patient.

The long-term failure of most leaders to place the right emphasis on loving care and to provide adequate guidance and support to frontline caregivers has caused a cascade of problems in caregiving. Indeed, when we look at the care *not* being given to hospital patients, it seems that we actually need to restate the obvious: The bedridden patient is a *human being* in need, not just a robot requiring a mechanical adjustment.

As we explore this matter further, you will discover what I have observed across a quarter-century of work in hospitals. When people become patients, they are rapidly marginalized by the system. Patient gowns and IV lines seem to signal that the patient has now become something less than a full-fledged human. The hospitalized ill are often referred to with a variety of demeaning sobriquets such as "the gall bladder in 5028" (person with gall bladder disease) or "the frequent flyer" (regular visitor to the ER) or "the screamer" (disoriented patient who groans a lot).

I have heard every one of the above terms used frequently in hospital settings. The use of terms like these not only marginalizes the ill person, but gives some caregivers the idea that they are permitted to degrade the patient by ignoring their requests and keeping them for hours on steel gurneys in cold hallways.

TRANSFORMING THE PATIENT GOWN INTO A CLOAK OF RESPECT

One of the most humiliating garments ever designed is the standard patient gown. How do you feel when you see someone in one of these outfits? It would be hard to keep a straight face if the person wearing it weren't so sick. These gowns are such a sign of degradation in American culture that in the movie "The Doctor," the senior physician played by William Hurt forces his residents to change into patient gowns so they can get a sense of how demeaning they are.

Take off all your clothes and put on one of these things. The likelihood is that you'll feel worse instead of better. In the Christian story, Jesus' captors sought to demean him by stripping him down to a simple cloth and pressing a crown of thorns onto his head. Patients who feel diminished by sprouting IVs and catheters can seem even more diminished by the simple cloth that drapes them. For ten years Susan Quintenz, a colleague of mine, and I attempted to determine a new design for the patient gown. We even sought advice from The Limited clothing stores in an effort to find a fashionable and dignified solution. Unfortunately, we never felt satisfied with any one choice, and we ended up thinking that multiple choices may be better than a one-size-fits-all option. Frankly, I may have been off track in trying to redesign the patient gown. The issue is really about how we treat patients more than it is about how they are dressed.

The solution is for healthcare leaders and doctors to begin to see the patient gown as a cloak of respect that represents a season of suffering for a human being. When we are in this season of suffering, we take on the gown of a patient. No one would wear one of these outfits if they weren't already diminished by illness. The patient gown must become a signal to all caregivers that here is a patient in need — a wounded person in need of a Samaritan — a fellow human in need of special respect.

From this moment on, may we commit to training ourselves to take this new view of patient gowns. From now on, they are cloaks that demand respect.

THE INVITATION OF HOSPITALITY

If there is any concept worth restoring to its original depth and evocative potential, it is the concept of hospitality. It...can deepen and broaden our insight in our relationships to our fellow human beings.[1]

— Henri Nouwen

Because hospitals were established as places of hospitality, we should consider, as Nouwen does, what "hospitality" means. When ill patients come for hospitalization, they are extending an invitation to us to help them through their season of suffering.

Nouwen writes, "Maybe the concept of hospitality can offer a new dimension to our understanding of a healing relationship."[2] The woman who comes to the hospital asking for help with the delivery of her baby is inviting us to share with her one of the most intimate and profound times of her life. Hospitality calls caregivers to respect and honor this invitation.

As in the Christian tradition, this is an inverted invitation, as the guest becomes the host and the host becomes the guest. Doctors and nurses are invited to be guests who are welcomed by the patient into her body and into the experience of her labor and birth. Like guests, they are expected to treat every element of the host with respect, and they can be grateful to the host for inviting them into this experience.

LOVING SERVICE *vs.* CUSTOMER SERVICE

It's time for a revelation. It's time for deep system transformation. The need for change cannot be met with fancy customer service programs aimed exclusively at "increasing patient satisfaction." The radical loving service referred to in these pages is something that must arise from two directions: 1) a critical new initiative from leaders and 2) a renewed commitment of caregivers to loving care. Hospital CEOs pay so much attention to the business needs of the hospital that they often forget to pay attention to the caregiver's needs. This situation needs to change — now! Patients are lying in waiting rooms at this moment waiting for help from harried caregivers. These caregivers need to be supported by leadership that is committed to giving them the help they need to get the job done.

Chuck Lauer is publisher of the most influential magazine in healthcare today, *Modern Healthcare*. In a column in his magazine he launched a well-intentioned attack on the world of hospital ERs by describing his own unsatisfactory experiences. He went through multiple encounters in two different hospitals during which he was kept waiting for ridiculous amounts of time and given rude and abrupt instructions. "My problem was with the customer service, or lack thereof, in ERs," Mr. Lauer writes. He describes the similar bad experience of a friend who is not only vice-chairman of a Fortune 500 company, but the chair of a hospital board. This friend chose to take time at his next board meeting to demand that things be changed. He is quoted as saying, "I recited my story and we had a lot of discussion on emergency rooms and people kept waiting much too long."

What can we suppose happened after this kind of high-level grousing? The publisher of a major healthcare magazine and the chair of a hospital board both complain about bad ER experiences, and around America, healthcare leaders read the article and nod their heads in agreement. They've had bad experiences, too. "What a shame," they may say. So is anything going to change? I've run hospitals for years and I can tell you the answer most likely is no. Hospital administrators are used to dodging around in situations like this. The likelihood is that the leadership at those hospitals has solemnly promised that they will "look into that." Translation? No change. But who will solve this problem if *they* do not?

America's healthcare systems, including its ERs, are incredibly resistant to change. It is false to think that a board chair's complaints will do anything more than affect his own personal care. He may be moved to the head of the line next time he comes in. Everyone else will be kept waiting and the system will creak on unchanged.

There are fundamental systemic obstacles to change. For example, in many hospitals, the Admitting department is separate from all other departments. The head of an ER may want the admitting clerk to adopt a more loving approach to patients, perhaps by saying to entering patients, "I'm sorry you're in pain, let me do this paperwork as quickly as possible" . . . but she can't approach the clerk because the clerk is not under her direction. The head of the ER is supposed to go to the head of Admitting to engineer even a change as simple as this one. But in a Healing Hospital, all departments would be on the same page and an important change like this would flow naturally.

The reason we must go beyond customer service to loving service is that customer service only addresses cosmetic issues, while loving service reaches

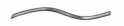

far deeper. Any hospital can bump up its patient satisfaction scores temporarily with a smile campaign. But ultimately, campaigns like this breed cynicism among employees, who may feel they're being treated like children. After a "smile campaign" presentation in another hospital, two employees were overheard in the hallway saying to each other sarcastically, "Now you be sure and smile!"

In the same hospital, a daughter reported that she said to a nurse, "Maybe this is a stupid question, but could you tell me a little about what the experience will be like as my mother goes through cancer treatment?" The nurse said to her, "You're right, that is a stupid question." Smile campaigns and customer service cosmetics will never solve problematic interactions like this. Loving service offers critical guidance to both managers and frontline staff as they learn how kindness, compassion, and respect are essential ingredients of clinical excellence. Loving service is based on trust, and it relies upon the maturity of partners to determine how they can live out their truest beliefs about caring for others.

Basic change in the treatment of patients and staff members won't come quickly with just a couple of stern orders from the executive office. It *begins* with a decision in the boardroom by committed executives and concerned board members and doctors who have decided the system can be changed and that the change will start in the organization where they serve. After that initial decision the change can take a period of months and years, and it involves everything from hiring and orientation to fundamental changes in basic systems.

The healing approach is about core change in the culture of hospital organizations. If, together, we begin this work today, our brothers and sisters lying in hospitals across America will begin to experience the kind of care we should all receive, whether we're chair of the board or a poor person in off the street. Then we will experience the sea change so desperately needed in American healthcare. And only then will we be able to say that we are truly living out the missions we proclaim.

HOW SIMPLE LANGUAGE CHANGES CAN AFFIRM HUMANITY

To love means to open ourselves to the negative as well as the positive — to grief, sorrow, and disappointment as well as to joy, fulfillment, and an intensity of consciousness we did not know was possible before.[3]

— Dr. Rollo May

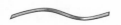

Dr. May's words remind us that we live in a world of paradox in which we are constantly finding ourselves acting in ways different from what we believe. We say we will love someone no matter what, and then find ourselves drawing away at the first sign things are turning negative. Dr. May also writes, "Hate is not the opposite of love, apathy is." When we are confronted with the pain of another, one of the classic ways to cope is to become indifferent — to say to ourselves that we don't really care. We become like children who are not invited to a birthday party who, to deal with the pain of rejection, say, "I didn't want to come to your birthday party anyway." This kind of indifference is the fabric of the shield so many caregivers put up between themselves and patients. It's not hatred. It's apathy that stems from the mistaken notion that if we use caring words with a person in pain, we will be unable to stay as objective as we need to be.

Millions of encounters happen in America's hospitals every day. They involve a vast crowd of patient transporters, radiology technologists, dieticians, nurse's assistants, billing clerks, social workers, physical therapists, lab technicians, housekeepers, pharmacists, phlebotomists, and a dwindling number of registered nurses. What can leaders do to enrich the texture of these encounters with a whole new approach to caring? All hospital mission statements call for caring, and yet caring attitudes are remarkably infrequent in most hospitals.

Let's look again at the hard world called the Emergency department. When we come into an ER with a pain in our side, *why* does the admitting clerk ask us for our name and insurance card instead of using words that express concern for our condition? It's because she or he has been told that this is her job. This admitting clerk would surely describe herself as a loving person. So, by the way, would her supervisor. With proper management support and training, this person could be encouraged to say something that demonstrates she truly sees the patient before her as a human being. This could be something like: *"I'm so sorry to see you're in pain. Let me get this information as quickly as possible."* This comment takes only a few seconds but is dramatically more humane than the typical admitting clerk mantra: "Name. Address. Insurance Card …"

Other types of language changes can be implemented by hospital leaders. To foster a culture of loving care, employees in a Healing Hospital are called *partners*. The simple language change may not seem important and it is not legally significant. But language always affects thinking. The lan-

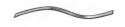

guage of partnership encourages frontline staff to think of themselves as working with leaders rather than for them.

THREE SYMBOLS OF LOVING SERVICE

Loving care has a long and beautiful tradition in human history. In these pages the heritage of loving care is symbolized by the image of a Golden Thread, which is also a symbol of faith in God. It represents the positive tradition of healing versus the negative tradition of transaction-based behavior.

A second symbol, a pair of intersecting circles, signifies the merging of love and need in the Sacred Encounter, which is the fundamental relationship between caregiver and patient. This symbol also signifies hope — the hope that comes into our hearts when we experience loving encounters.

The third symbol, a red heart, signifies the nature of the Servant's Heart. It also symbolizes love and is love's greatest expression. This expression, although it specifically references the heart, assumes the full involvement of our best thought processes. Loving care is not loving if it fails to engage the best skills and competency of caregivers.

These three images represent the trinity of values that signify the way in which radical loving care can be described and understood. We call it *radical* care because the call here is not for random thoughtful gestures but for a *continuous* chain of loving care — kindness and skill from every caregiver (including leaders) to *every* patient and to one another.

Loving care consists of more than simple kindnesses. Loving care also means *skill, competency,* and effective *stewardship* of resources. If your doctor gives you precise medical care but in a way that is disrespectful, this is clearly *not* loving. Neither is it loving if your doctor is kind to you but gives you sloppy and inappropriate medical carer. The Sacred Work of the Healing Hospital does not abandon technology or ignore business forces. Rather, the Healing Hospital joins loving care and clinical care in a new and exciting vision of clinical excellence — Healing Care — a new vision for all of America's hospitals. The Healing Hospital represents a vision of

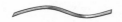

true excellence built on the most important principle of human existence — loving one another.

HOW A HEALING HOSPITAL CREATES POWERFUL RESULTS

Fortunately, a Healing Hospital also produces results. How would you like to be part of a hospital that: 1) is in the top one percent in patient satisfaction, 2) has outstanding employee morale, 3) has low turnover, 4) has exceptional clinical care, 5) has a score of 98 from the Joint Commission on Accreditation of Healthcare Organizations, 6) demonstrates good financial performance, and 7) is characterized by an extraordinary chain of continuous loving care?

Does this sound like somebody's image of a healthcare utopia? Or like some kind of hokey sales pitch connected to a toll-free number? In fact, this is the kind of hospital all leaders should be trying to create. I have personally seen at least two examples of this kind of hospital — Riverside Methodist in Columbus, Ohio, and Baptist Hospital in Nashville, Tennessee. And there are others, like Saint Charles in Bend, Oregon, and the Dalles Hospital, also in Oregon. These are the kinds of hospitals every patient and every caregiver wants. We call them Healing Hospitals. With genuine commitment, it is possible to create these kinds of hospitals and other healthcare organizations all across America.

As every company CEO knows, goodwill alone will not generate success if it is left to the shifting winds of randomness. Effective *systems* are crucial to the success of a Healing Hospital. The importance of placing love at the center is that love creates an environment in which the employee partners become passionate about creating systems that will work because they desire the best possible outcomes for patients.

For example, the Care Partner program at Baptist, developed under the direction of Perri Lynn White, R.N., offers Care Companions to each patient over 65. This program is not only about being kind to seniors — it helps the hospital as well as the patients. Patient falls among the elderly are one of the biggest causes of morbidity and mortality in this age group. The Care Partners program will reduce the number of these falls. A reduction in falls would also lead to a reduction in lawsuits — another concrete outcome. In addition, the Care Partner program is, logically, an effective way to build patient loyalty in this age group and their families.

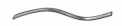

The Sacred Encounter, where love intersects with patient or partner need, is the best expression of loving service. This concept has the effect of creating a sense of meaning and purpose for frontline caregivers. Many types of hospital work can be perceived as drudgery unless they are infused with the meaningful energy of sacred encounters. The housekeeper in our story *could* think of her work as just mopping floors. For many, this kind of work could quickly become boring and work performance might fall. But the housekeeper thinks of herself as a caregiver, not a floor mopper. Redefining her work brings a whole new hopeful energy to the work, and productivity rises.

Hiring for a Servant's Heart is not just about attracting and retaining kind-hearted people. Hiring people who are committed to serving others above themselves is also the most effective way to reduce turnover and improve general employee satisfaction. Satisfied employees are likely to mean satisfied patients. They are also much more likely to be more productive, make fewer medication errors, and give a genuine commitment to the organization.

Each of us does our work every day based on a particular kind of energy. We want to act out of love, but we may be acting out of fear. We may go to work primarily because we are afraid of our boss, afraid of not having enough money, afraid of failure.

The call of loving service is a call to act out of love, not fear. A culture of loving service creates an environment that we want to enter each workday. It is a place where we would never be afraid of our boss because our boss is our partner who is working to support us in our jobs. In a Healing Hospital, work is done out of a passion to care for others. Nurses don't choose the nursing profession to become rich. The best nurses choose caregiving out of a passion to serve. Leaders have a responsibility to support nurses in this service by providing the best environment possible.

PREREQUISITES FOR THE HEALING HOSPITAL

There are at least three prerequisites that must be met in order for the work of a Healing Hospital to be accomplished. First, there must be a *deep commitment* from top leadership to focus on staff training around loving care. Second, there must be significant changes in *systems and structures;* this is one reason we refer to the work as *radical* loving care. Third, we must consider that people learn best not from long lists of instructions, but through *dialogue and respectful inquiry.*

1. Leadership Commitment

Things will never change until leaders change. This begins with commitment. If you are a senior leader, what is the legacy you plan to leave? The only way to do the job right and to leave a meaningful legacy is to commit to truly living out the mission of your organization, and to do it more effectively than did your predecessors.

2. Changing Systems and Structures

Consider, again, the Emergency department. Patients don't come to the hospital to be registered, they come to be treated. Not-for-profit hospitals should not be turning down patients, so there is no need to demand an insurance card before treatment is given. In order to improve loving care in the Emergency department, it is wise to move the admitting function away from the front desk. The first person a patient sees should be a skilled caregiver who can either begin treatment directly or guide the patient to someone who can.

Such system changes should be made in all other departments as well. Employee partners who are trained to give loving service need to be supported in this care. The wrong systems and structures may interfere with and even defeat this objective. A change in systems and structures signals to frontline staff that the organization is serious about supporting loving service.

3. Teaching through Dialogue and Inquiry, Stories, and Piloting

In the fifth century B.C.E., Socrates taught with a method of dialogue and inquiry that today bears his name. The Socratic Method emphasizes teaching with a pattern of questioning. One of the most beautiful characteristics of this method is that it places trust in the inherent intelligence of each student. With Socratic teaching, there is a presumption that each student has the ability to figure out answers on his or her own if the right questions are asked. And students are better able to remember what they have learned if they have had to think through the way in which they answer these questions.

The Socratic Method is unparalleled. Extensive leadership experience has taught me that the best teaching methods use this approach of dialogue and inquiry. Didactic teaching, the kind where a speaker reads data to an audience, is to be avoided or at least minimized in a Healing Hospital because it is so incredibly ineffective. Most people learn best by doing and by teaching themselves, not by sitting and listening to long lectures. Give heavy emphasis to the process of dialogue and inquiry in order to advance your healing work. Stories, or teaching parables, are strong ways to teach as well, and they can be an important part of the teaching dialogue.

A companion to these learning/teaching processes is the active process of *piloting*. Ideas can be developed and piloted in small settings over brief periods of time. This minimizes risk and resource commitment and maximizes the chance to test an idea. It is critical, however, that a failed pilot not lead to automatic abandonment of the plan. Give the staff a chance to engage in dialogue about how to improve the pilot and consider re-piloting the new model instead of giving up. Remember that pilots can be done with time as well as size limitations. Successful piloting is a good quick way to gain affirmation for the job and to cut the task down to bite-sized pieces. As with the Socratic Method, partners engaged in piloting may learn from a leader who suggests a program, but they will teach themselves and learn from their peers as well.

With these three prerequisites, the vision of a Healing Hospital is eminently achievable. Consider the case of Nashville's Baptist Hospital System — an organization that recovered from a state of crisis in 1998 to become the first Healing Hospital in the country.

BAPTIST'S TRIPLE TORNADOS OF '98: ADVANCING LOVING CARE IN THE FACE OF A CRISIS

In April of 1998, I visited Nashville, Tennessee, as a candidate for President and CEO of the newly announced combination of Baptist and Saint Thomas Hospital Systems. The combination would create a six-hospital system in middle Tennessee, including two of the largest hospitals in Nashville. Shortly after my arrival at a hotel in town there was a weather warning, and all hotel guests were ordered to a basement level. Soon after that, several tornados ripped through the area. One of them struck parts of the campus of Baptist Hospital, causing about $300,000 worth of damage.

Soon a second kind of tornado struck Nashville. This one was organizational. A couple of weeks after my interview, the two organizations announced that the merger was off and no CEO would be needed since there would be no combined entity to run. The merger had blown apart.

The next chapter in this story emerged when I was asked to serve as

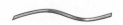

President and CEO of The Baptist Hospital System upon the retirement of the previous longtime Baptist head. I accepted. On October 1, 1998, I took the helm as the new leader of the System. At the time it was a four-and-one-half–hospital integrated delivery system (one hospital was owned jointly with Saint Thomas). The organization had interests in Health Maintenance Organizations (HMOs), including a TENNCARE Insurance Company, a Preferred Provider Organization (PPO), and over one hundred physician practices. It was also the principal healthcare sponsor of the Tennessee Titans National Football League team and the Nashville Predators National Hockey League franchise.

I had been advised that the system bottom line was predicted to be a gain of about 10 million dollars. A departing leader told me pointedly, "Erie, one thing I can tell you is that there are no skeletons in the closet." I thought back on this last line many times as I discovered what looked like lots of trouble everywhere.

Then the third tornado struck. Again it was the organizational kind of weather strike, and again, it caused major damage. One week after I began as the new President and CEO, the Chief Financial Officer came to tell me that several major adjustments were necessary. It turned out to be much worse than I could have imagined. The real bottom line of the system for Fiscal Year 1998 would show a staggering loss of $73 million dollars on an operating budget of about $400 million!

The actual tornado that hit Nashville did far less damage to Baptist Hospital than did the financial tornado. What do you, as a leader, do when you discover that the organization you've just started to run is 83 million dollars worse off than what you thought when you started? What happens to mission and values in the middle of such a situation? The turnaround of 1998–2001 at Baptist is a clear indication that one of the best ways to lead an organization out of tough times is to use the Healing Hospital approach.

THE HEALING HOSPITAL

A Healing Hospital is a place characterized by thousands of small and wonderful things and a few big ones. At the center is love. My colleagues and I believe that the mission and values of the Healing Hospital should remain as strong during any emergency as they are during day-to-day activities.

The Healing Hospital is a concept that, more than anything else, supports a strong culture of caring. It expresses the deep passion of both

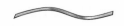

patients and caregivers. This is a passion in the human cry of the suffering patient. It is a cry for help, and for love. And it is also the silent call emanating from the eyes of caregivers who seek real support from leadership in their desire to respond to that human cry.

The hearts of most organizations do not seem to be awakened to this need for caring. Sadly, many hospitals, particularly for-profit systems, act too often out of desire for economic gain and fear of lawsuits. We believe the focus should be on clinical excellence and loving care and only secondarily on driving the organization toward financial success, even — especially — during times of financial or other crisis.

Some of the things that characterize a Healing Hospital and Radical Loving Care are: 1) every single employee partner treats patients with loving care — we call this the continuous chain of caring, 2) every single leader treats staff with love and respect, 3) all hiring is done with a focus on finding people who have a Servant's Heart, 4) orientation and staff reviews are focused on a balanced evaluation of both results and values, 5) people who cannot support this approach are respectfully removed from the organization.

It all begins with leadership.

THE LEADERSHIP OF PARTNERSHIP

We must always be tough-minded and tenderhearted.
— Dr. Martin Luther King, Jr.

My old high school football coach used to shout and scream at us. His drill-sergeant style intimidated me, and I didn't like it. His motivational talks consisted of tirades during which he would bellow something like: "I want you jerks to get out there and grind those guys into the ground. I mean I want you to KILL them." I wish I could tell you that this approach didn't work. The truth is, the varsity team on which I played had two straight undefeated seasons.

Why does this drill-sergeant style work? Well, it works in football for the same reason it works in the military — the goal of the leader is to goad followers to do something *violent*. I do believe that football players and soldiers can be motivated with more of a partnership style, but my point here is that the threatening style of leadership can be effective if the goal is violence.

It is to be hoped that hospital leaders have a different goal. The Healing

Hospital approach requires a leadership of partnership. Can you imagine a healthcare CEO gathering nurses together and yelling at them: "I want you to get out there right now and CARE!" People cannot effectively be ordered to "be loving." Love can flourish in many of us, however, if we are in an environment that encourages it.

Most important is that leaders in a Healing Hospital need to think of their primary work as supporting the frontline staff. Since CEOs don't take care of patients, their job is take care of the staff — *to take care of the people who take care of people.*

> *The CEO's job is to take care of the people who take care of people.*

A partner-oriented leadership style that is openly respectful of the views of others is the kind in which trust and caring will flourish. The best ideas will not only bubble up in this kind of atmosphere, but they will be heard! Theodore Roosevelt said, "People ask the difference between a leader and a boss. The leader leads, and the boss drives." Too many hospital leaders still think they are hard-driving football coaches or army generals instead of leaders ministering to caregivers.

The single exception to the partner approach can occur temporarily in cases of emergency. When emergency strikes, command/control approaches are not only expected but also welcomed. From a leader's standpoint, emergencies are the exception not the rule, and command-style leadership should likewise be an exception.

The rest of the time, partnership should be the watchword and the action style. Command/control is an effective style in military models when the goal, in wartime, is to do a pattern of things that are fundamentally violent — such as attacking and killing an enemy. Aspects of command/control can be seen in hospitals in environments like operating rooms and classic emergency-room traumas. Most of the time, however, the operating room should be a relatively calm place, as should the Emergency department. Both run best when doctors and nurses work together as partners.

But even in the face of emergencies, loving leadership is important. Martin Luther King's words about being simultaneously "tough-minded and tenderhearted" ring especially true here. An example of the importance of this balance emerges from a painful story in which I took part many years ago.

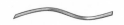

THE ROLE OF LOVING LEADERSHIP IN EMERGENCIES

The hour is striking so close above me,
So clear and sharp,
That all my senses ring with it.
I feel it now: there's a power in me
To grasp and give shape to my world.
— Rainer Maria Rilke

December 30, 1983 — "Erie, one of our employees has just been murdered down the hallway."

There are dates, and moments within those dates, that so deeply scar our memories that they can never be forgotten. On December 30,1983, I had been serving as President of Riverside Methodist Hospital for about six months. I was sitting in my office at 4:45 p.m. It was supposed to be the holiday hiatus between Christmas and New Year's, yet my wonderful secretary, Elaine Jenkins, was also there, as were several other executives.

Suddenly Dr. Ed Bope, a family physician on staff at Riverside, burst into my office looking as pale as his lab coat. In the calm voice of a professional he said to me, "Erie, one of our employees has just been murdered — in the Research Lab down the hallway. I think it just happened."

News of murder — murder just a few dozen feet away — made that hour strike very close above me in a way that was as clear and sharp as I have ever felt. It is at times like that when the senses are open in the way that Rilke described. It is also a time when you grasp to give shape to your world — a world that seems suddenly chaotic. "Are you sure she's dead?" I asked, wondering if there was still a chance for this doctor to save her.

"There was no need to check," he said. "When you see her, you'll understand why."

Hospitals, of course, are built for medical emergencies. Doctors and nurses train for them. Hospital presidents and their staffs train for how to handle emergencies like plane crashes, fires, and bomb threats. In large, complex hospitals like Riverside Methodist, patients die every day. But there had been no training on how to deal with a murder in the hospital.

The Research Laboratory was only about 100 feet down the hallway from my office. In my three years as a prosecutor I had never seen anything like what I was about to confront.

When I saw her, my first thought was that the body of our poor, innocent Lab partner looked like a mannequin. She lay face down on the floor of the Research Laboratory in a large pool of her own blood. Dr. Bope said she looked so pale, so blue, so without life because she was "exsanguinated": all the blood had left her body. She had suffered numerous stab wounds and her throat had been slashed, leaving her skin completely drained of the color that blood would give to it. To add to the nightmarish scene, she had been "hog-tied" — hands and feet pulled up and tied behind her with rope.

The horror of such a scene is the kind of shock that can make it difficult to act. Yet in crisis, the spirit of loving leadership must remain steady. The tough side of a leader needs to take command of such a situation. At the same time, the tender side needs to stay in touch with the sadness of a life lost.

I still had the responsibility to direct a 1000-bed hospital through this tragedy. With the help of my advisers and using what I had learned in other less-horrible situations, I would have to find a way through.

Since the murder looked recent, there was a continuing risk to the rest of the hospital and its 700 or so patients and staff and visitors. I wished at that second that I could hit a button and lock every door in the vast building in order to catch the murderer. But there were no less than fifty-six exits to the hospital, all of them equipped with roll bars for easy opening. The police had to be notified, but as soon as they were called, the media would know. This would create a new level of chaos because patients and families of patients would hear that someone had been murdered in the same building where they were bedridden. And yet the family needed to be contacted, and some message had to be given to the frontline staff.

We called the police and posted a security guard at the door to protect the scene. I was grateful to see our outstanding General Counsel, Frank Pandora, coming down the hallway. I left Frank in charge of the scene and went back to my office to set up a command center. Frank turned out to be a terrific support throughout this ordeal.

Interestingly, another key member of our leadership team left the hospital in the middle of the crisis. When I asked him later where he had been, he said, "Well, I left because I figured that this situation didn't have much to do with the area for which I am responsible." Fortunately, the rest of the senior staff did not follow this cold and narrow approach.

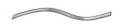

But one of the senior staff members who did stay crumbled in the face of the bad news. When I returned to my office and verified that one of our partners had been murdered, this executive put his head in his hands and said hysterically, "Oh no! Oh no! What are we going to do? What are we going to do?" I told him to go to his office, that he could call his wife but no one else, and that he should stay in his office until he calmed down. Then I closed the door to his office. *Leaders do not have the luxury of giving way to hysteria in the midst of a crisis.* All energy and attention needs to be focused on how to serve others most effectively, not how to deal with our own personal worries.

It was a special gift to have the steady and competent advice of Marilyn Marr, our senior communications executive. Marilyn gave excellent counsel throughout this crisis — which was particularly impressive since she was a friend of our murdered partner. One of the first things she said was that we needed to compose an immediate short message to all of the staff explaining honestly what had happened and providing them with reinforcement and encouragement.

We began to compose the message. Then something even more stunning happened.

David Whyte, in his life-changing book *The Heart Aroused,* retells the ancient story of Beowulf so that we can apply it to our own lives. After Beowulf kills the dreaded monster Grendl, Beowulf and his friends believe they have conquered the beast. In the midst of their complacency, even worse news is brought to them. Grendl's mother has now appeared and she is an even fiercer and more threatening monster than Grendl. That is what happened at Riverside. We learned we were facing a more frightening beast.

The police had arrived and told us they believed the murderer or murderers were no longer in the building. By now it was about quarter past five and the hospital was wrapped in midwinter cold and darkness. Christmas decorations still adorned the halls. The Lab partner's lifeless body still lay on the floor of the Research Laboratory. As Elaine called members of the staff to my office to receive the message we had composed, I went about setting up a three-part command center to get a headstart before the press arrived — one part for dealing with the press, one for supporting the families, and one to run the hospital.

Suddenly the terrifying ghost of Grendl's mother appeared through news on the telephone line. What is worse than one murder? With one murder, we had a somewhat contained situation. But what if there were more? Frank Pandora phoned me from the murder site to tell me: "The

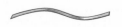

police just found a second body."

The first murder was both horrifying and heartbreaking, but after the report of the second murder, I was more than twice as alarmed about the immediate welfare of our patients and staff. In spite of police assurances, the discovery of a second body created the clear possibility that the murderer was roaming the hospital killing people.

The second body had been discovered in a refrigerated room used by the Research Lab. This poor woman, another partner from the Laboratory named Patricia Matix, had been killed in the same way as the first. The police told us that the assailant had limited his murderous actions to the Research Lab and had then fled.

As we continued to set up the command centers and notify the families, the press arrived in a rush and were directed to the hospital's boardroom. Then came the next challenge to healing leadership. Marilyn said we needed to make a statement to the press right away. I encouraged *her* to do exactly that. She told me *I* needed to give the statement.

She was right, of course. But what do you say in the middle of such horror? I thought about my goal, as goals always help to define content when something important has to be communicated. My goal, as president of the hospital, was to respond caringly to the deaths and to simultaneously keep the hospital running smoothly in the face of potential panic. We all know that you can't calm people down by simply saying, "Don't panic!" This was clearly a time for the best possible combination of tough-minded/tender-hearted action.

I entered a wall of white lights and noise as I walked out to talk to the press. This scene is common on many news broadcasts, but I had never been on the microphone side of the cameras in an emergency situation. When the environment is flooded with blazing lights and cameras are whirring and snapping away and voices are calling out from the other side of the light, it is disorienting at a time when strong focus is critical. Someone once told me that the best thing to do in circumstances like this is to remember that it's not about you — it's about other people and the organization. Here is roughly what I said, as best as I can recall twenty years later:

> "I'm Erie Chapman, President and CEO of Riverside Methodist Hospital. Tonight we are devastated to report that two of our employee partners have been murdered. On behalf of the hospital, I want to extend our deepest sympathies to their families

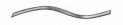

and friends. This is a hard loss for all of us here at Riverside and we mourn the passing of these two wonderful servants.

"These murders took place in the Research Laboratory of the hospital, and we believe this tragedy is isolated to that part of the hospital. Accordingly, the rest of the hospital is running smoothly and patient care is not being affected in any way. I want to thank our staff for continuing to provide wonderful care though this difficult time. They are demonstrating the best spirit of professionalism and will continue to take excellent care of our patients and each other.

"As you can see, this is now a police matter, and I am referring all further inquiries to the police."

This turned out to be a successful communication because: 1) it helped calm down anxious staff, patients, and the public about the safety and stability of the hospital, 2) it adequately expressed our heartfelt sympathies, and 3) it truthfully isolated the murders as a "police matter" rather than a "hospital matter."

The hospital continued running normally for the rest of that horrible night.

Thank God there were no more murders at Riverside. We hired off-duty police officers to augment our security force and began a complete overhaul of security operations in our facility. We also held a memorial service for the two fallen members of our staff and later erected two memorial fountains in their honor.

The rest of this story unfolded in a way that is often sensationalized in television movies. In fact, the story of the capture of the murderers was made into a movie.[4] Three years after the hospital murders, William Matix (Patricia's husband) and a partner were captured in a bloody shootout with the FBI in Florida. Matix and his partner, both of whom had been on a murder spree through the south, and two FBI agents were killed. Matix, now dead, could never be formally convicted of involvement in his wife's homicide, but it seems highly likely that this murderous man and his partner were responsible for the murders of two innocent partners at Riverside on the second-to-the-last day of 1983.

IF LOVE FAILS AT HIGH LEVELS

Things can turn out badly if a leader in a crisis does not maintain the tough-minded–tenderhearted balance. The tough mind needs to make the good decisions, but people do not want to follow a leader who does not show his or her human side.

Although the traumatic event was hypothetical, not actual, we can learn from an answer given in the 1988 Presidential debates between George Bush and Michael Dukakis. CNN's Bernard Shaw posed a question to Governor Dukakis about his position on capital punishment. He asked what the Governor would do if an intruder broke in and raped and killed his wife. The Governor answered with a cool, clinical analysis that described the need to contact the appropriate authorities and follow the appropriate procedures.

Somehow, whether because of overcoaching or the pressure of the debates, this otherwise compassionate person failed to say anything about how he would feel about this kind of attack on the woman he loved. He never said he'd be upset or broken-hearted. He remained so cool and calm that he came across as uncaring. That evening and the next day, he was roundly criticized in the press for his failure to express any of his feelings. As you know, he also subsequently lost the election.

LOVING LEADERSHIP ESPECIALLY IN TOUGH TIMES

One of the most common excuses I hear for failure to carry forward the mission of caring is that it's not practical to do so when things are either in a state of emergency or when there are financial pressures. I hope this book will make clear that loving leadership is called for on *all* occasions, *especially* in tough times.

We ask a lot of our leaders. Most of all, we ask them to magically maintain the right balance in the most difficult of times. And we are inclined to be remarkably hard on them if they don't. This is why any of us who aspire to leadership need to constantly practice King's tough-minded/tenderhearted balance in every part of our lives.

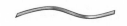

Chapter 2

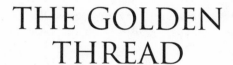

THE GOLDEN
THREAD

We all are healers who can reach out to offer health, and we all are patients in constant need of help. Only this realization can keep professionals from becoming distant technicians and those in need of care from feeling used or manipulated.

— Henri Nouwen[5]

We are all healers, and we are all patients. As both healers and patients, a Golden Thread of loving care connects us all. In western civilization, hospitals were founded in the fourth and fifth centuries by churches for the purpose of offering hospitality to people suffering in illness. A Golden Thread links America's hospitals of today with those hospitals of old. Indeed, this thread of loving care extends from the present back to the first instance in human history when one of our forebears cried out in pain and a fellow human offered loving help in answer to that cry.

When did one human first reach out to another in need? Clearly, human encounters based on loving acts are ancient. But the truth is, we can respond to any cry for help in at least three ways: we can ignore it, we can take advantage of the other person's weakness, or we can respond to the cry for help with love. The parable of the Good Samaritan[6] powerfully illustrates this choice because the Samaritan responds after others have passed by. Further, he offers sustained help. He takes the man to an inn for care and leaves money with the innkeeper for follow-up care. He even offers to provide more help and to return later. His love, therefore, is open-ended and without limits.

Through modern psychology, we have learned a scientific basis for something the ancients believed as well — that love is essential to life itself. In contemporary hospitals, we have learned that *babies who are fed but not touched will lose weight and die*. They die because they have been deprived of human contact — of the power of human love from one person to another.

For centuries, a cruel and effective way of punishing human beings has been to place them in solitary confinement or to otherwise shun them from a community. Isolation works as a form of punishment for the simple reason that human beings need loving relationships with others in order to live healthy, meaningful lives.

Love is essential to life itself

A basic truth of human existence is that we all need love. A Healing Hospital is built on the ancient tradition that love is at the center of healing. The Golden Thread of healing has fallen to the ground in many hospitals where loving care has been shoved to the sidelines, replaced by the new twin idols of technology and business.

ROBOTS *VS.* HUMANS

He's more machine now than a man; twisted and evil.
— Obi-wan Kenobi speaking of Darth Vader in *Star Wars*[7]

One of the ways to characterize evil is to imagine something that kills people in a way completely devoid of human feeling or conscience. Was this what Hitler was — a human-like "thing" who ordered the murder of millions, without remorse? Was he merely a masquerade of a human being, with a human appearance draped over a killing machine? This extreme reference helps us imagine the real differences between a robot and a human.

What *are* the differences? This question is more pressing now than it has ever been in history. Most of the body is now astonishingly replaceable; from the tops of our heads to the tips of our toes. Plastic surgeons can add hair, remove wrinkles, replace our noses, and provide us with new ears, new

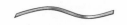

chins, and new lips. Orthopedists can replace our knees and our hips. Even our hearts are replaceable — either with the heart of a transplant donor or with a mechanical heart.

What about our brains? Computers can perform many memory and analytical thinking functions far more effectively than can the human brain. Computers can even play chess against international chess masters. It is not difficult to imagine a circumstance in which computer chips would be implanted in our heads to send us data and help us perform analytic activities. Could even our brains be replaceable?

Meanwhile, human cloning is not far away. And the Human Genome Project offers astounding potential for other advances that will likely protect us further from disease and extend the lives of our bodies.

What's left that makes us uniquely human and distinguishes us from robots? Four centuries ago, Descartes, with his famous statement "Cogito ergo sum" (I think, therefore I am), said our thinking ability was what proved our existence. Now it seems more likely that a better statement would be, "I love, and therefore I am." A robot has no ability to love — or to form anything we would describe as a genuine relationship. We would also say that a robot has no soul. Perhaps it's a further improvement on Descartes' state-

> *I have a soul, and therefore I am.*

ment to say, "I have a soul, and therefore I am." Clearly, my body is mostly replaceable, and even my thinking ability can be significantly replicated in many respects by a computer. But my ability to interpret ideas that are meaningful to me cannot be replicated.

The late Michelle Jackson, who was a colleague of mine at Vanderbilt Divinity School, had a couple of chronic illnesses that sapped her energy right up to the moment of her untimely death at age thirty-eight. She said once to me, "I hurt, therefore I am." Of course other animals experience pain as well. But humans are capable of a multi-layered and complex experience of pain — an experience that goes far beyond their physical reaction. This human complexity is something the medical establishment needs to explore more deeply and seek to understand. A better comprehension of the complexity of human pain can inform us about what we need to do to address the deeper needs of patients in our hospitals. When people become patients, they are entitled to even more human understanding. Instead, they often receive less.

We currently rely on the instinctive loving behaviors of housekeepers and nurses and other caregivers. Loving service in a Healing Hospital calls

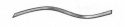

us to a deeper study of the field of the human reaction to pain. This enables us to learn more systematic methods of addressing these more complex levels of agony.

It may still be true that I think, therefore I am. But it is also true that I hurt, therefore I am, I have a soul, therefore I am, and I love, therefore I am. Each of these statements shouts the humanity in each of us, and the need for special attention from caregivers when we are made more vulnerable by illness — when we, as people, are suddenly referred to as patients.

HOUSES *VS.* HOMES

Consider the differences between a house and a home. A house is a structure built so that people can inhabit it. For a house to become a home primarily requires the imponderable elements, those whose value, unlike the value of indoor plumbing or a sturdy roof, cannot easily be defined. In nearly four decades of marriage, I never thought any new house I inhabited became a home until my wife put in place the unique and special things that create our sense of family. These elements are so precious that they defy description, yet I'm sure that you understand the critical distinction between a house and a home.

Indeed, every adult and most children know the difference between a house and a home, just as all of us have a sense of the difference between robots and humans. Yet in our age the distinction needs to be discussed again, because the differences can be very hard to describe and are, ultimately, impossible to quantify. How much, exactly, do you love the first home you ever lived in? How much, exactly, do you love your family? Even though these things are not quantifiable, they are endlessly important.

ORDINARY HOSPITALS *VS.* HEALING HOSPITALS

Lacking positive myths to guide him, many a sensitive contemporary man finds only the model of the machine beckoning him from every side to make himself over into its image.

— Dr. Rollo May[8]

Inside these contrasts — between robots and humans, houses and homes — are the ingredients that are crucial to understanding why Radical Loving Care is required to convert an ordinary hospital into a Healing Hospital. As Dr. May suggests, we need positive myths to guide us. And it

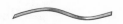

is love that underpins all positive beliefs. A true home is suffused with love; so is a Healing Hospital. So much depends on each of us accepting that it is possible for our hospitals to offer loving care in a continuous chain. It sounds radical, but it is doable. And even if there are rare breaks in this chain, the effort to create the chain will dramatically improve the world of acute medical care.

Hospitals need to be more than just places of physical care — of "robot-repair." When faith-based Christian hospitals consult their tradition, they will rediscover that Jesus did not come to earth to perform healing miracles on the flesh. His primary mission was to provide healing for the spirit with faith, hope, and "the greatest of these . . . love." For example, he made a request to the lepers he had healed to keep silent and not tell anyone of the miracle he had performed on them. It seems logical to assume that Jesus was concerned that too much attention on his healing miracles of the flesh would draw our attention away from his efforts to heal our souls.

THINKING ABOUT PATIENTS

The concept of the Golden Thread can be used in any hospital system. The way to do so is to explore the particular healing tradition of a given hospital and then to consecrate it with a renewed commitment and a new pattern of loving behaviors. A good place to start is with an honest evaluation of the attitudes that may exist among leaders and frontline caregivers. For example, how are patients viewed? This question is more challenging then it may seem.

A century ago Sigmund Freud taught that each of us comes to a given situation prepared to see it in a particular way, based on the preconceived images we have learned. Peter Senge picked up this concept and articulated it further by labeling some of our preconceived ideas "mental models." The models cause us to see other people through a particular lens of interpretation. Dr. Richard Glenn discusses the concept of mental models in his helpful book *Transform*.[9]

A caregiver may view a patient through a mental model of "the patient as stranger." But so long as we think of patients as strangers, we will have difficulty extending to them the love they deserve. In faith-based systems, if we can think of each person as a child of God, then this means that all of us are brothers and sisters. This is a mental model that can free caregivers to extend to each patient, and to each other, the loving kindness that releases the power of healing care.

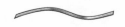

Caregivers may also subconsciously perceive patients as weaker (and therefore lesser) human beings because of their illness, a mental picture that may be unfortunately supported by the humiliating design of patient gowns. As suggested in Chapter 1, caregivers need to develop a new mental model that allows them to consider the patient gown as a cloak worthy of special respect.

The Golden Thread calls us to place the advances of science in balance with the demands of the human spirit. We are called to attend to both the heart and the head. This means we must look again at the relationships our staff has with the vulnerable human beings we call patients.

Recall the story of the housekeeper and the old man. The story may seem small. Yet it is through thousands of small stories like this one that the Sacred Encounter is advanced. Inside that little story, the human cry of the old man is met not by a cold transactional response but by love. It can be a keynote story in a Healing Hospital because: 1) it signals the willingness of a housekeeper to be a caregiver, 2) it highlights the chance every employee partner has to redefine his or her job, 3) it signals to supervisors what is valued in the organization, and 4) it offers an example of a front-line employee partner showing her Servant's Heart and engaging in a Sacred Encounter. When the housekeeper took the hand of the sick old man in hers, she carried forward the Golden Thread of loving, healing care.

Inside this story is the trinity of images that characterize a Healing Hospital — The Golden Thread, The Sacred Encounter, and the Servant's Heart. For a hospital to be truly healing, the Golden Thread must be continuous. Each partner must be engaged every day and night in encounters like this.

In words that echo the spirit of the Golden Thread, Chief Seattle is thought to have said in his famous speech of 1854:

> You must teach your children . . . that all things are connected like the blood that unites one family. Whatever befalls the earth befalls the sons of the earth. Man did not weave the web of life; he is merely a strand in it. Whatever he does to the web, he does to himself.

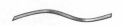

Chapter 3

FIVE CHALLENGES TO A
HEALING HOSPITAL

*People can be made to feel better by many things, including sympathy
and kindness . . .*

— Arnold Relman, M.D., professor emeritus,
Harvard Medical School[10]

THE NEED TO EDUCATE HEARTS AS WELL AS MINDS

Why do America's healthcare leaders perpetuate the myth that hospitals are places of loving care? Perhaps because this once was true. The myth continues to be advanced because hospitals are *supposed* to be places of caring and because certain caregivers actually continue to practice caring in the face of dehumanizing crosscurrents. Unfortunately, these caregivers are in the minority because, increasingly, work environments tend to emphasize efficiency over kindness as if the two were mutually exclusive.

The truth is that places that actively practice loving care have better outcomes. In fact, with results like increased patient and employee satisfaction, reduced turnover, and improved financial performance, why isn't everyone rushing to create a Healing Hospital? Indeed, every hospital that can do this should do it. Great outcomes at hospitals driven by loving service, like Saint Charles in Bend, Oregon, Baptist in Nashville, and, in the 1980s and '90s, Riverside Methodist in Columbus and Beth Israel in Boston, offer proof that hospitals can be both loving and successful.

And there is an encouraging new wave of hospitals that are rethinking their mission work and how to apply it at the front lines. These outstanding hospitals and hospital systems have made the courageous decision to seek change on the front lines. They are pioneers, and the rest of America's hospitals need to get on board or risk continued mission failure! Among the early leaders are Dennis Vonderfecht, President and CEO of Mountain States Health System in Johnson City, Tennessee, where the Healing Hospital model is being implemented; George Mikitarian, President & CEO, Parrish Medical Center, Titusville, Florida; Lloyd Dean, President and CEO, Catholic Health West; and Bonnie Phipps, CEO of Saint Joseph's Health System in Atlanta.

Still, those who accept the task of establishing a Healing Hospital approach are faced with several challenges. It cannot be emphasized enough that missions are not truly effective until there is *clear evidence of change at the front lines!* The kind of patient comments and letters that count are the kind I received at Nashville Baptist after the Healing Hospital initiative had been implemented. These are the comments and letters that said, "not only was my stay outstanding, but *every single partner* I encountered treated me with loving care."

Veteran leaders know what they're up against, but this should not cause them to hesitate. The patient-centered mission of the organization is at stake. The Healing Hospital challenges appear in five characteristics of modern healthcare whose influence constantly tests the mission of loving care:
1. Technology and Prescription Drugs
2. Business Factors
3. Bureaucracy
4. Cynicism
5. Failed Leadership

1. Technology and Drugs: Deus ex machina?

"I'm talking about perhaps even being able to reverse the aging process, turning the time clock off . . . We are developing digital technologies that have an output to the biotech area . . . We'll have the ability to turn on and turn off

certain genes to promote health. "[11]

— Dr. James Canton, futurist

Reverse aging? Turn the time clock *off?* Perhaps Dr. Canton, a noted healthcare futurist, got a little carried away, but well-known healthcare experts like him are now making these kinds of startling statements. The thrilling advances of medical technology and magic-bullet drugs have proceeded so quickly that we have become enchanted by the possibilities. The *deus ex machina* in Greek and Roman plays was a god who was introduced by means of a crane in order to suddenly solve all problems, and we have unwittingly begun to look at technology as a kind of *deus ex machina* — as if, somehow, God were now contained in robotics and MRIs instead of within the human soul. In Nouwen's words, technology has "depersonalized the interpersonal aspects of the healing professions."[12]

Given a choice, all of us would prefer laproscopic gall bladder surgery with a one-day recovery to old-time scalpel surgery with a six-week recovery. And who of us, facing general surgery, would decline a dose of Valium to calm our anxiety? In the year 2003, surgery performed on us by doctors in distant cities directing robots is considered to be a real possibility *within five years.* The lure of the pharmaceutical company's newest hot drug is virtually irresistible. But these exciting new developments have become so dominant that we are losing sight of other healing essentials such as the loving-care approach and the idea that body, mind, and spirit are unified.

We can, in part, blame René Descartes for the notion that body and mind are separate, a view he set forth in the early 17th century. We can only blame ourselves for staying stuck in the Cartesian construct. The notion of splitting our thought process away from our physical function seems so logical today that it is almost second nature. In the West African culture, however, traditional thinking is quite different, and tribal ceremonies reinforce the belief that earth, mind, and body are all one. In one ceremony, the names of ancestors are spoken out loud. As each name is recited, water is poured on a plant and the word Ashe (pronounced Ash-ay) is spoken. As I understand it, this is to emphasize recognition of an ancestor who has gone back to the earth and whose memory must be honored by how we live our lives. This way of thinking of the body, mind, and spirit as unified

> *In our society techno-cratic streamlining has depersonalized the interpersonal aspects of the healing professions.*
> — Henri Nouwen

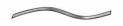

and one helps people raised in this tradition to think more holistically.

The western tradition emphasizes separation and division. Medical treatment for disorders of the body is seen as the province of the physician. Treatment for disorders of the mind is reserved for psychiatrists and psychologists. Treatment of the spirit, for patients in hospitals, is often reserved primarily for the hospital chaplain or other cleric. Sadly, the notion that each of us is an integrated spiritual being who should be treated as a whole person is almost foreign to western medical training.

In a funny little film from more than sixty years ago called *Susan and God*[13] the lead character, played by Joan Crawford, says, "What's the use of all these mechanical inventions if they don't make everybody happy?" We need modern technology for effective medical care, but what exactly is the value of this technology in hospitals if patients are not also being treated with kindness and caring? And what about the numerous challenges brought by technologies that often prolong the lives of people who are living a very low-quality existence? Does technology really always make things better for us? Are we yielding too much power to shiny new machines?

Every year, *U.S. News and World Report* publishes a list of what they call "America's Best Hospitals." The 2003 edition trumpeted "Exclusive Rankings of Top Medical Care"[14] on the cover of the magazine. The criteria for these selections are heavily weighted toward research and teaching facilities with a high emphasis on technology services and academic reputation. Actual patient satisfaction is not taken into consideration in the survey. While it is sometimes difficult to track the full quality of a patient's experience, national organizations like NRC/Picker and Press-Ganey have made strong efforts to trace this information in America's hospitals. NRC/Picker has a particularly strong record of being able to customize testing tools for patient and employee satisfaction so as to give healthcare leaders the most reliable possible testing tools. This organization's annual conference, typically in Boston, is one of the finest gatherings in the country for hospitals truly interested in being patient-centered.

> *Sadly, the notion that each of us is an integrated spiritual being that should be treated as a whole person is almost foreign to western medical training.*

Not surprisingly, and of very deep concern, large research hospitals often have low patient satisfaction. It's time for America to begin noticing hospitals where both clinical excellence and patient satisfaction are high.

We in the Healing Hospital movement are obviously not saying that new drugs should be resisted, but that the use of drugs and technology needs to be balanced by recognizing the role of loving care for hospitalized patients.

It is clear that the importance of loving care has receded in direct proportion to the advance of technology and scientific learning. It is as if we have subconsciously assumed that if we can fix something with a machine, there is no longer a need for the loving touch — the touch that was so vital to us in our first weeks of life.

The latest technology may be enchanting, but who of us would like to be attended in our most agonizing moments of pain — or in our dying moments of life — by a robot? The wires, tubes, monitors, and electronic beeps that currently surround dying patients in America's intensive care units suggest that the tentacles of technology already have us in their grip.

2. Business and Profits

"Is it really about technology? No, no, it's about increasing market share. It's about increasing sales. The battle for the future is about the battle for your customers."

— Dr. James Canton, healthcare futurist[15]

In case we have any doubts about how cynical the healthcare world has become, we need only note the words of Dr. Canton. He simply articulates publicly what many others discuss behind closed doors in healthcare meetings. Are the great advances in technology and medicine about helping patients? "No, no, it's about increasing market share. It's about increasing sales." Frontline caregivers may feel differently, but many leaders have turned their eyes away from loving care and toward profits.

How we spend our money is a reflection of what we value. Recent reports provided by the American Hospital Association reflect that the expense budget for America's licensed hospitals is now in the neighborhood of half a *trillion* dollars each year. How much of this money would we estimate has been spent in advancing loving *care* for patients versus technology-based cures? And how much has been squandered on things connected to neither?

The charitable hospitals of the past have become sophisticated high-revenue business corporations in the present. In addition, high-population states like Texas and Florida are dominated by for-profit hospitals owned by publicly traded companies. The risk of shareholder interests taking

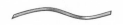

precedence over patient concerns is real. The likelihood that millions of dollars have been diverted away from direct patient care is evidenced in the claims of scandal that have plagued for-profit healthcare giants like HCA, HealthSouth, and Tenet.

The advent of Medicare and Medicaid in 1966 ensured that hospitals would begin receiving payment for care that had often gone uncompensated in the past. Government money also guaranteed that revenues flowing through hospitals would rise sharply. No one can shrink the business behemoth that the American medical-industrial complex has become. In 2001, expenditures for America's registered hospitals alone exceeded 426 billion dollars.[16] The high percentage of the GNP (now over 13%)[17] committed to healthcare suggests how highly health is valued by the American people.

Yet the advance of business issues, along with a parallel but lesser advance of unions into America's charitable hospitals, seems to have driven out the idea that America's caregivers see healthcare as a calling. This has frustrated the nurturing of the concept of the Servant's Heart in medical care.

Although ignored and underappreciated, the Servant's Heart still beats. It is up to America's healthcare leaders to reawaken the loving spirit in America's caregivers by providing work environments that nourish this spirit instead of frustrating it. Leaders must interpose themselves between caregivers and the dollar demons that threaten them. It should not be the responsibility of a beleaguered frontline nurse to solve the problems of a patient's HMO.

3. Bureaucracy: Prisons and Patient Gowns

"Visiting hours are now over. Will all visitors please leave the hospital."
— Announcement on hospital P.A. system

"Visiting hours are now over. All visitors must leave the premises."
— Announcement on prison P.A. system

America's largest and often most highly ranked hospitals are a nearly hopeless labyrinth of confusing hallways and preoccupied employees. When I began working in hospitals in 1975, I had just completed three years as a federal prosecuting attorney with the United States Department of Justice. When I entered the world of hospitals I noticed that the process of a patient's admission into a hospital bore a striking resemblance to the process of imprisonment.

Consider what happens to us when we become patients. Our clothes are taken and replaced with a patient gown, a garment that is at least as humiliating as an orange prison uniform. Then our name and patient number are wrapped around our wrists. We are wheeled into semi-private rooms with complete strangers. The rooms feel more public than semi-private — the door is not only unlocked but is entered dozens of times a day at the convenience of caregivers. Visiting hours restrict friends and family, and in spite of the well-intentioned nature of these rules, they can leave both patients and employees feeling like hostages. Even worse, hospital partners cast into a system like this can subconsciously begin treating patients as if they had lost their ability to think or were small children. The tone of voice can become condescending — laced with the language of parental control.

> *America's most highly ranked hospitals are a nearly hopeless labyrinth of confusing hallways and preoccupied employees.*

My father-in-law, Dr. Leif Lokvam, a physician felled by a stroke toward the end of his long life, experienced this when he went from being the doctor to being the patient. Comments from caregivers, who used to address him as "doctor," went like this (in a tone as if speaking to a little child): "How are we, Leif? Have we eaten our dinner yet? We're going to eat our dinner now, aren't we?" My father-in-law, although aphasic (unable to speak) was otherwise in complete command of his mental abilities. His aphasic state and advanced age somehow seemed to give his caregivers the mistaken impression that he had lost his mind as well as his speech. Accordingly, he was unintentionally treated as a small child instead of as a mature, thinking adult.

None of these employees means to be disrespectful. It is the world of bureaucracy mixed with misunderstanding that has cast them in this role.

> *The monotony of my daily work makes me*
> *Wonder whether I am alive, or why.*
> *But let me be a loving craftsman with purpose,*
> *And my energy will be boundless.*

A common characteristic of bureaucracies is the assembly-line nature of many of the jobs. Such work can beat down workers as surely as any actual assembly line, especially if the worker sees no point to his or her job.

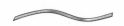

Hospital employees are not only asked to do repetitive work, but to do it as if they were robots instead of people.

This cycle of repetitive empty-seeming work can be broken. The repetitive process may be essential, but the repetition need not be meaningless. In fact, it can be infused with meaning, as illustrated by the inspiring story of cafeteria cashier Lois Powers (see page 61). A craftsman may engage in numerous repetitive acts, yet for him or her, the acts are meaningful as part of a creation. The work of a hospital caregiver can be like that of a pianist who plays the same sequence of notes in a repetitive pattern yet creates something beautiful, and who is motivated to repeat the repetitive work by the beauty of the outcome and its effect on the listener.

Caregivers can sometimes see the effects of their work on patients. But what about the information systems technologist or the person in the kitchen making dozens of salads? What do they see? What about the patient transporter who is taking your mother or mine from her room down to radiology? These partners may feel lost and ignored in the middle of the healthcare machine. The low pay level accorded to these positions may reinforce the sense of disconnection.

Money and bureaucracy can buffet high motives like a hurricane and cause caregivers to withdraw into a shell of indifference. None of us wants to have concern for profits take precedence over concern for patients. Yet the siren call of money can drown out the cry of the old man from the patient room down the hall, and the crush of bureaucratic demand may stamp out feelings of love.

When we embrace technology, we seek to direct it for the cure of our bodies. None of us intends for it to take over our souls as well. Yet there is an ever-present risk that we will surrender completely to one or all of the above forces — to the enchantment of technology, to the lure of business profits, and to the lazy thoughtlessness of bureaucracy.

4. Cynicism

"Don't ever tell anybody anything. If you do, you start missing everybody."
— Holden Caulfield[18]

The character of Holden Caulfield, in J.D. Salinger's *Catcher in the Rye*, was the ultimate cynic. The whole world seemed dark and phony to him. Yet from underneath this cynicism, he revealed the caring heart that most cynics have buried within them. *Don't ever tell anybody anything because this*

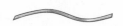

means you'll start missing everybody and this is painful. This is a caring heart slammed shut to protect it from the slings and arrows of life. The biggest reason people become cynics is that they don't want the pain that goes with being tricked. They've been tricked before, probably starting when they were six or seven years old, and they've vowed that they will use their cynicism as a shield to protect them from being tricked again. Some carry this so far that they automatically doubt everything. As a result, the cynic is deaf to the occasional person who is genuinely loving and caring.

Although cynicism is often toxic, some skepticism can be good. Cynicism can be a damaging cultural phenomenon, passed like a contagion, but skepticism, like constructive criticism, can provide a healthy counterbalance to lofty and impractical thinking. In general, many people, particularly trained professionals, are skeptical about the power of love in the patient care process. In fact, a wide-ranging crowd of skeptics either doubts or directly opposes the role of love in medical care.

Unfortunately, this skepticism has become cynicism enshrined in the culture of numerous medical schools, poisoning some nursing schools, and tainting many research centers where love is disdained as non-scientific and, therefore, irrelevant — if the subject even comes up. Love is not part of the evidence-based model of medicine — partly because love does not respond well to metrics.

The core problem with the western model of medicine is described effectively by Drs. Moore and Komras in their outstanding book *Patient-Focused Healing*.[19] Therein, the authors refer to "the subtle difference between curing and healing." They emphasize accurately that "Whereas curing focuses on the disease or injury, healing focuses on the person experiencing the disease or injury . . . When healing is the goal, the definition of success is expanded to include what the patient has learned and how well the patient is able to cope even though complete curing may not be possible." The authors emphasize that healing is multi-dimensional and therefore takes into account emotional and spiritual considerations as well as physical.

Frankly, this is all just so much common sense, except for the small problem that this kind of common sense is rare in hospitals. American medical care, in its obsessive focus on caring for a particular diseased part of a person, displays an astonishing ability to ignore the whole person being treated. Consider, again, the cynical view taken of love. In the American medical model, love seems like a "nice thing" but not an *essential* thing to physical recovery. In truth, there's no question that a broken leg can heal

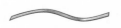

without an ounce of loving care. Yet a leg, broken or healed, only *matters* because it is part of a human being. A leg can be healed with science. A human being can only be healed with love. As Teddy Kennedy, Jr., said about his childhood hospitalization for bone cancer, "All my doctors ever asked me was: How was my *leg?* Not one of my doctors ever asked how *I* was."[20] As a result, he left the hospital somewhat cured of his cancer (although without a leg), yet bitter and dismayed by the failure of his doctors to recognize his humanity.

Why is this important? Who cares if doctors focus only on the disease and not the person? What is the responsibility of caregivers to integrate love with physical care? Put aside, for a moment, the prosaic example of a broken leg and consider, instead, the horrifying image of a woman who has been raped. What if this patient was given strictly "medical" care? What if her bruises and cuts were treated and issues of her emotional and spiritual trauma were completely ignored? Shockingly, this sort of situation may actually still occur in some of America's hospitals. But most hospitals would not think of releasing such a patient without appropriate and kind attention to the whole person. And if we attend to the whole person in cases like rape, why don't we do the same with every patient? Every patient has needs that go beyond the physical, and medical care should recognize and attend to those needs insofar as they may touch on effective healing for the whole patient.

In fact, the reason caregivers and the hospitals that employ them should take responsibility for loving care is threefold: 1) humans are complex beings who need love, 2) through their mission statements, hospitals hold out to the public that loving care is important, and 3) in faith-based hospitals, the standard is even higher since love is supposed to be at the center of every faith.

5. Failed Leadership: A Golden Opportunity to Convert Houses of Technology into Homes of Healing

A physician shall be dedicated to providing competent medical care, with compassion and respect for human dignity and rights.[21]

Principle #1
American Medical Association Principles of Medical Ethics

The first principle of the AMA Principles of Medical Ethics emphasizes not only competency but also compassion. Yet there has been a decline in the role of loving care in hospitals over the past half-century. That decline is *a failure of hospital leadership,* of both lay and physician leaders. Doctors and hospital CEOs have a responsibility to advance compassionate care and to ensure that it is offered on the front lines. Regrettably, I must certainly count myself among leaders who, too many times in the past, missed an opportunity to place loving care at the head of the agenda. The whole thing sometimes seemed too hard to achieve and too amorphous. Converting a hospital to a model of loving care does not lend itself to a Power Point Presentation as easily as does, say, an annual budget.

What happens to frontline staff people when they feel more like assembly-line workers in an auto plant than caregivers in a hospital? Rollo May addressed this matter brilliantly in his 1967 book *Psychology and the Human Dilemma*: ". . . when people feel their insignificance as individual persons, they also suffer an undermining of their sense of human responsibility."[22] This is the reason that inspired leadership that affirms the frontline staff creates greater productivity, and mechanical, demeaning leadership causes both lower productivity and less loving care.

One of the most important things leaders and physicians do is set the agenda for what is discussed in the organizations where they serve. For any leaders reading these words, here is your opportunity to change everything in your organization, starting immediately. This is your opportunity to move loving care to the top of the agenda. At your next staff meeting, ask your staff where they think loving care should be ranked. Ask them to formulate plans for how they would advance this work effectively at the front lines.

This can begin a cascade of change through the culture of your organization. Imagine if this question began to race around your hospital: *How can we go about giving loving care more effectively?* Don't be deterred by resistance based on the so-called greater amount of time it takes to give such care. As we have seen, it may not take more time at all — it may mean simply using the time caregivers have in different ways. Remember, you, as leader, needn't have all the answers. In fact, it's better if you don't — since the answers need to come from those who are directly engaged in caregiving. The golden opportunity is before us. It only remains for us to seize it and pursue it with complete passion and endless persistence! Healthcare leaders and physicians need to educate *their* hearts as well as *their* minds. Both groups must guide our hospitals toward being homes

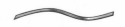

for the ill, not simply houses of technology.

The great, unfinished business of healthcare is not curing, but healing. Technology, business forces, bureaucracy, and cynicism are advancing as relentlessly as the cloned helpers in *The Sorcerer's Apprentice.*[23] These forces threaten to steal what remains of the soul of American healthcare. What is needed now is not so much a revolution as a revelation.

There is a deep need to rediscover the caring angel in each of us — the same one who guided the hands of the first loving caregivers — and to restore that angel to its place on the throne of healthcare. There is a parallel need for leaders to identify and support frontline caregivers — to lift up the concept of the Servant's Heart — and to rediscover the critical importance of the interaction of love with need in meaningful Sacred Encounters.

BALANCE AND CONSISTENCY: LOVE FOR THOSE IN THE SHADOWS

The moral test of a society is how that society treats those who are in the dawn of life — the children; those who are in the twilight of life — the elderly; and those who are in the shadow of life — the sick, the needy, and the handicapped.

— Hubert H. Humphrey

Former Vice President Humphrey (under Lyndon Johnson) eloquently described the state of illness as being "in the shadow of life." This is why the Healing Hospital concept was created. People in this shadow need consistent love as well as competent technical help. The goal here is not to cast aside technology, throw away drugs, and refuse Medicare reimbursement. The challenge is to restore equilibrium. The American healthcare system is not so much broken as it is dangerously unbalanced. The adjustment it needs is dramatic and deeply significant.

The bad news is that it will take a massive effort to restore the role of loving care to its rightful place as the dominant theme in medical care. The good news is that the distinctive feature of our humanity is our need for, and ability to give, love. As this core truth is revealed, love will rise up like a candle in a dark room, filling every corner with its brilliance.

It is startling and tragic to see how difficult it is to convince people of

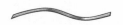

the obvious need for the restoration of love to the center of the healthcare paradigm. Hundreds of hospitals carry the image of the Cross or the Star of David. Yet in many of these hospitals, religious imagery seems like a quaint relic. The same kinds of forces that have split mind and body seem to have split our work away from our faith.

The American healthcare system is…dangerously unbalanced.

Hospitals with a religious tradition are obviously not the same as churches. But hospitals that hold themselves out as faith-based have a responsibility to be who they say they are. Presumably, this means they have a high standard of responsibility to live out the tenets of their faith by the active practice of loving care.

In hospitals with no religious tradition, caring is still held up as important in speeches but is not lived out in practice. Efforts at secular humanism are often no match for the forces of technology, business, and bureaucracy. Loving care has thus far been unable to defeat the cynical view that human beings are machines and hospitals are gigantic repair shops. Yet love may still return to its rightful place at the center.

As we seek to reestablish loving care, the questions turn to the method of building a Healing Hospital. What are the methods, and how are they expressed? How does one go about "constructing" a whole new culture?

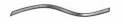

Chapter 4

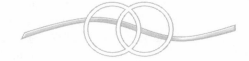

SACRED ENCOUNTERS, SACRED WORK

"I have some very bad news."

TWENTY-FOUR HOURS IN THE BABY INTENSIVE CARE UNIT

There are countless encounters between caregivers and patients in every hospital every day. In order to appreciate how sacred these encounters can be, we often need to be reminded that, in a hospital, life and death are each on the edge of happening suddenly and frequently — and pain is ever present. At Baptist Hospital, in an average twenty-four hours, two people will die and seventeen will be born. As I used to say regularly to new employee partners in orientation, "Today is the last day on earth for two people within these walls, and they are spending that last day with us. And today is also the first day on earth for seventeen people. They are spending it with us as well. What could be more sacred than to be with people on their first or last day on earth? And what could be more meaningful than to be present with them when they may be in their greatest pain or highest joy?"

Yet the magnificence of life and death and pain often overpowers front-

45

line caregivers. Perhaps the most eloquent description of what caregivers see each day comes in the form of a sort of journal entry written by a physician. Dr. Elizabeth Krueger is an exceptionally gifted neonatologist at Baptist Hospital with twenty years of experience. When she is on duty, she is medically responsible for as many as thirty babies in their earliest and most fragile state. She is the specially trained physician who cares for infants like the very tiny premature babies who used to die quickly, entering and leaving this earth within minutes of their birth. Medical advances and her own skills now enable her to save those babies on many occasions. But she is still accustomed to tragedy. As Nouwen says, "We are all healers who can reach out to offer health, and we are all patients in constant need of help." Dr. Krueger shares here a gripping and poignant picture of just one twenty-four-hour shift in her work life in what we can call the baby intensive care unit.

I arrive at the hospital to be on call for the next twenty-four hours. It is four days before Christmas. I will eat, sleep, and live in this very unusual mini-world with little access to windows or day/night cues. I will not relax. An alarm may sound at any second, signaling a life-threatening emergency. A phone might ring summoning me to disaster. I am used to this; the adrenaline stays at a constant low stress level in my blood. It can't possibly be good for me.

At home, I have not put up my Christmas tree, as I have been studying . . . My kids are to arrive home from school that day, while I am at work. I haven't seen them for three weeks. I feel like a bad mother.

I enter my office to unload my things. My partner walks in. "Sit down, I have some very bad news." I am used to bad news. But this was horrible news. The day before, when I had been on call, I had counseled a young couple getting ready to deliver a set of twenty-four-week twins. I liked them a lot. I told them all they needed to know. I told them that if all went well, over the next three months, we would all get to know each other very well and be like family. The delivery went great and the twins were off to a wonderful start. I was full of hope and optimism. That was yesterday.

But my partner is telling me that a "code" has just ended. It is not on the infants, but on their mother. She stood up in her hospital room to come visit her babies and she just died. She is only thirty. I walk into the nursery. Everyone is in tears. The care manager is a wreck. But there are babies to care for, including two little motherless ones.

The day proceeds calmly. The grieving family is making funeral arrangements. We look at these babies as though they have somehow become even more dangerously precious. Motherless children.

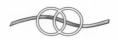

At about six that evening, after a quiet afternoon of reading in my office and doing paperwork, the phone rings. "They need you STAT in 3107. Something about a tumor." I run down the hallway, huffing and puffing, and arrive to find a vigorous, crying infant with a horrendous birth defect. From the anus to the umbilicus, the internal organs are inside out. Exstrophy of the bladder. I can't even say for sure if this is a boy or girl. I speak briefly to the parents: "Your baby has an abnormality of the bladder. I think she is a girl, but for now let's not say. We need to check her chromosomes to be sure. This is a problem that can be repaired." We will speak more after I get things stabilized. So I whisk away their little one, leaving them in their horror. They cannot even call relatives to say, "It's a girl."

After we medically stabilize this infant (IV, blood work, monitors) I return to the shattered parents. The chaplain comes with me. We spend some time talking about what the future holds: the different operative stages of repair and the likelihood of normal functioning in about half of these children. I even address the "why" — I don't know, an accident of nature, no one's fault. I am leaving as the chaplain asks them if they want to pray. They say yes. I ask if I can join in. We hold hands. The chaplain stays with them.

About midnight, things are settling down. A nurse tells me there is a new baby in normal nursery with Down syndrome. I have dealt with this many times, but I know the parents have not. Still, it is not a medical emergency. Their pediatrician can tell them in the morning. But the nurse says to me, "The mother knows something is wrong, won't you talk to her?"

How can I say no? The chaplain has gone home. I go out to the room of this couple that I have never seen before and will never see again, and I shatter their world. I sit for a long time, just watching them absorb the enormity of what has happened to them. I cannot just state the facts and depart. I try very hard to be present and calm. I stay to answer the questions that continue to surface. They do not need to be alone. I ask if they want the chaplain to be called in. They do not. I leave much later. I feel like kicking a hole in the wall. I overhear the nurses at the station being critical of me. "You'd think the neonatologist would go talk to them." They do not know I have been in the room with them for the last hour.

It is now about 2 A.M. I try to sleep but can't. Fortunately, the rest of the night is quiet. I make rounds on all the babies the next morning, and leave the hospital about noon. I get home to find my house a sweet mess with teenagers moved back in for Christmas. We decorate the tree. I am drained. I spend a lot of the afternoon under a blanket on the couch. I wish I were a better mother. My kids, unfortunately, are used to this.

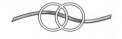

In the emotional wave that follows a story like this, it may be best to sit quietly for a time to reflect on the life of this servant and the agony and joy that make up her work. We can honor her and her story by being present to it for a moment, just as she struggled to be present in each of her three encounters.

One truth that bursts instantly from this eloquent story is the pain of perfectionism that edges the voice of this committed servant. Why is it that great servants are so often hard on themselves? Is it because they set higher standards? Is it because they have tuned themselves so carefully to the needs of others that they are overwhelmed? Saint Vincent de Paul, one of the great servants of history, said once about himself that he thought he was a "miserable wretch."

We read this story and want to applaud this doctor for her heroic commitment to helping others across the last twenty-four hours, not to mention the last twenty years. Yet all she can do is reflect on what a bad mother she is for being present, on this occasion, to suffering babies instead of her own grown children. Is she also thinking she should be back at the hospital when she is home? The double worry of trying to be all things to all people is the chronic challenge of any committed person. We want this doctor to forgive herself for not being home on time. Of course we forgive her — although we may wonder why the subject even comes up, since there is nothing to forgive. The challenge is not about our forgiveness, but about her accepting the grace of her own forgiveness. It's easy for us to sermonize about how each of us must love ourselves, but it's terribly hard for many capable people to live out this advice and accept God's grace.

Eleanor Roosevelt wrote, "Friendship with oneself is all-important because without it one cannot be friends with anyone else in the world." These words remind us that loving care begins with the self and with God. Love of God leads to love of self and love of self, as a child of God, leads to love of others. Our bodies and our minds are both of this world. At our creation, our spirits descend into our bodies from God. One thing that enables servants to love others is their appreciation that the personality is not the person. It is the spirit of another that draws our love.

Clearly, we don't have to like other people in order to love them. Each of us is filled with imperfections. If we only liked perfect people, we wouldn't like anyone. Loving ourselves does not mean we don't attempt to

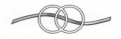

overcome our imperfections, but it does mean we accept these imperfections without shame. Parker Palmer writes, "Depression is the ultimate state of disconnection . . . between one's self-image and public mask."[24] Professional caregivers are constantly at risk for this disconnection because they may feel they have to offer such a perfect mask to the public. We need to provide opportunities for caregivers to gain relief from the exhausting masquerading that our society requires of professionals. And we need to help them develop new and healthier mental pictures about their work.

Meanwhile, Dr. Krueger's story is so rich with the music of Sacred Encounters that it can inform us on many additional levels. Dr. Krueger shares three types of patient encounters that happen in just one of her shifts. But first, in the opening two paragraphs, we receive a sharply defined picture of her multiple worlds. On one side, a "very unusual mini-world with little access to windows and day and night cues." On the other, at home, a place where "I have not put up my Christmas tree" even though "my kids are to arrive home that day." How many of us, caught up in our perfectionist desire to please the complex multiple worlds in which we live, find ourselves both stretched and stressed. As the doctor says, clinically diagnosing her own environment, "It can't possibly be good for me." Yet she chooses to continue her service anyway. The world of a true servant is never ideal. That is part of the reason for the service — to change that world.

We are all healers and we are all patients in constant need of help, says Nouwen. He also says that only the realization that we are both healers and patients "can keep professionals from becoming distant technicians and those in need of care from feeling used or manipulated." Our early images of doctors as healers may show them as professionals with answers, not "patients" in constant need of help. Because this physician has the courage to be more honest than most, we can see in Dr. Krueger both healer and patient in need.

What about the home life of healers? I remember the first time I saw my fourth grade school teacher in a setting other than school. As a nine-year-old, I was startled by the notion that she had a life outside the classroom. It had just never dawned on me that Ms. Croak would go shopping in the Woolworth's store just like little me. As adults, we often subconsciously forget that the nurses and doctors who are caring for our critically ill mother or son have private lives away from work — lives that may be severely strained by the nature of their healing work.

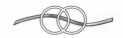

"Sit down, I have some bad news," a partner tells Dr. Krueger as she begins her first Sacred Encounter. Yes, doctors are accustomed to bad news. Family doctors deal with plenty of it. There is the need to tell the patient that the tests came back showing cancer or AIDS or heart disease. But intensive care doctors and nurses sit each day alongside death, sewing garments of healing around their patients to hold him back awhile.

The constant challenge is whether the doctor can sustain the balance between intense mental concentration and the need to stay open to genuine human feelings. In the first encounter, Dr. Krueger enters the story of a young couple on the threshold of exquisite joy. On the other side of that threshold is the risk their twins will die. Or perhaps, like the ancient story of Beowulf, there is an even worse tragedy that could rise up like Grendl's mother.

One anticipates death's victory over twenty-four-week twins. His theft of their apparently healthy thirty-year-old mother is obviously a terrible shock — even to Dr. Krueger. But she describes the scene by telling of the reactions of the care manager and the other nurses. Everyone else is in tears. What about her? "...there are babies to care for, including two little motherless ones."

> *Intensive care doctors and nurses sit each day alongside death sewing garments of healing around their patients to hold him back awhile.*

The need for doctors to hold back their feelings in the presence of emergencies is not unlike the need for leaders to keep their heads in the face of other kinds of emergencies like the murders earlier described. The full expression of their grief may not be a luxury caregivers can indulge in at the moment. This doctor has already entered the gold zone of a Sacred Encounter. She has already gotten to know the couple and has counseled them. She has even allowed herself to "like them a lot." Other nurses were in tears because they had chosen to enter that gold zone as well. They chose to care.

There is always risk as well as joy in the gold zone of Sacred Encounters, and it requires courage to enter. As nurse leader Debi Villines, R.N., says, "We can't turn our back on our patients' pain."[25] Unfortunately, many caregivers do turn their backs on the pain of others. Perhaps they are feeling overwhelmed and undersupported. Or perhaps they have lost courage and are trying to seal themselves off from the pain of patients to avoid any risk of pain to themselves. In so doing, they block the patient from receiving the compassion that is so desperately needed at times of crisis.

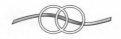

For this caring doctor, though, the day is far from over. She carries the Golden Thread of healing in her hands as she enters her second pattern of Sacred Encounters with a baby with a "horrendous birth defect." You and I have a choice about whether we even want to keep reading since she has warned us in advance that it will be hard. But this caregiver has no choice. In fact, she not only has to hear and see the horrendous problem, whatever it is, but she knows she will have to determine how to treat it — and to deal with the parents.

After the pain of the sudden death of a young mother, the doctor now faces the challenge of trying to correct a cruel surprise from nature. But before that challenge, the Sacred Encounter calls her to join the chaplain in beginning the process of helping heal these "shattered parents." This baby about whom they have harbored such hope now faces a lifetime of physical and emotional hardship — and so do they. The idea of stepping forward and actually asking permission to join a circle of prayer would seem awkward and even "unprofessional" to some doctors. But Dr. Krueger understands that Sacred Encounters like these can be a helpful part of healing grieving parents and she asks permission to participate. Sacred Encounters are characterized by unconditional love of the kind this doctor seeks to provide. None of us can do this perfectly all the time — or maybe ever. Yet the call of Radical Loving Care is that we strive to do our best.

In her third Sacred Encounter, the doctor offers loving support to parents of a baby with Down syndrome. She has never seen these people before and knows she will never see them again. But instead of brushing the parents off on the pediatrician or instead of a cursory report to the shattered mother and father and a quick exit, she strives "to be present and calm" with these wounded people for a full hour. She understands that they are patients as well.

Beyond her kindness, what else is this physician thinking and feeling about these triple nightmares? She tells us. "I feel like kicking a hole in the wall." This caregiver is not trying to be a hero to us in her story. She is willing to be vulnerable enough to let us see her human side. Storybook heroes are never honest enough to admit they feel like kicking walls. And perhaps we can understand the anger that wells up in her over the human suffering she sees each day and how it makes her want to rail against the irrationality of it all by doing something irrational herself. On top of all this, instead of being thanked for her work, she is criticized unthinkingly by nurses behind her back.

There is no harder gift to give than unconditional love. And it is so crit-

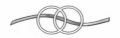

ical to understand that at every moment in this twenty-four-hour journey, this doctor could have chosen the more distant and less engaged pathway. She could have forsaken the rich forest of loving care and chosen the concrete highway of transactional exchanges. The language of doctors traveling that concrete highway would be very different in these different encounters. The death of the thirty-year-old mother might have been met with a brief, "Too bad, didn't really know her. Whose fault was it that she died? How are the other patients doing?" The encounter with the birth defect could be treated as simply a problem requiring surgical correction, and the parents could have been routed to other caregivers. Clearly, Dr. Krueger could have dodged the third encounter by simply telling the nurses that the pediatrician would handle it in the morning. But each time, this doctor elected to stay engaged — at considerable emotional and physical cost to her.

Finally, she approaches the end of her shift and then returns to her family.

It is now about 2 A.M. I try to sleep but can't . . . I make rounds on all the babies the next morning, and leave the hospital about noon. I get home to find my house a sweet mess with teenagers moved back in for Christmas. We decorate the tree. I am drained. I spend a lot of the afternoon under a blanket on the couch. I wish I were a better mother. My kids, unfortunately, are use to this.

What do we ask of our caregivers in a Healing Hospital? If we are challenging them to be consistently loving across twenty-four-hour shifts like this one, what will they have left for their families when they arrive home? This is why the support of leadership for caregivers is so crucial. Leaders have plenty of challenges of their own, but typically, leaders don't care for patients. Instead, leaders need to take care of the people who take care of people. They need to love frontline caregivers and to show this love by constantly honoring and affirming their work and creating cascades of support groups — Care Circles — that will provide a chance for healers to be healed. In order to be instruments of love, caregivers need to receive love as well. This will better enable the Dr. Kruegers of this world to be the kind of caregivers we would like for our hospitalized family members — and it may even help them to be better mothers or fathers as well.

In just one twenty-four-hour period, Dr. Krueger was baptized in the tears and pain of three different families, a sacred experience she has been

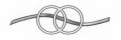

through many times because she is so loving and open. She has immersed herself in what my colleague Tim Glover calls the fragrant intimacy that comes when we choose to enter another's suffering. She also has many opportunities to share the joy of her patients. What is so significant about her expression of Radical Loving Care is her courageous willingness to keep her heart open while simultaneously offering her best skills as a physician. This is the model we seek for every caregiver in a Healing Hospital.

WORK AS A CALLING

We are instruments of divine love . . . We were created in God's image, in the image of love, and our goal is to grow more fully into that image by loving each other and the world in concrete . . . ways . . . Our task is to become aware of God's presence . . . We are called to see differently — and then to live differently . . .

— Sallie McFague, Ph.D.[26]

Vocatus atque non vocatus
Deus aderit

Called or Not Called, God is Present

The great psychologist Carl Jung kept the above statement over his front door throughout his career. This phrase, found in the Latin writings of the 15th-century theologian Erasmus, is fascinating when contrasted with an earlier version of it found in a Delphic Oracle to the Lacedonians: "Yes, the gods will be present, but in what form and to what purpose?"

The God of Erasmus is not only singular and all-powerful, but also clear and present in all things. So the question is not whether there is a God, but *in what form* do we experience God, and what are God's purposes for us?

In the Christian tradition, Jesus reveals to us that God is love. Christians, Jews, and Moslems — anyone who believes in love — are called not to create love, but to *discover a love that is already there*. This suggests that faith-based hospitals have a special responsibility to be who they say

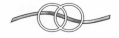

they are. The simple act of the housekeeper reveals: 1) that she is open to hearing the need of another and 2) that she is open to responding to that need with unconditional love. The more complex acts of Dr. Krueger reveal exactly the same thing. These caregivers are pursuing their work as a calling.

"Called or not called, God (Love) is present." These words speak a fundamental truth — that every single one of us working in a faith-based hospital is called to reveal God's love to every patient and every partner with whom we work. This calling is no small task — but it is a task worth the effort. Our effort to meet this challenge provides the ultimate meaning for our work.

As Professor McFague suggests, we are called to "see differently — and then to live differently." In so many ways, our society and our daily work teach against the pathway of love and toward the pathway of material gain through endless transactions. We who choose the life of caregiving must not only learn to see differently, but to listen differently as well — so that we may hear the human cry of need.

Every so often, someone will "discover" an image that seems to capture the imagination of certain segments of the world population. An example of this is a recent reported sighting of an image of the Virgin Mary in the third-floor window at Milton Hospital in Massachusetts. "The phenomenon is basically the human ability to see pictures out of randomness. There are trillions of these and they just wait for someone to notice them," says Joe Nickell, a senior research fellow at the committee for the Scientific Investigation of Claims of the Paranormal.[27] Whether Mr. Nickell is right or not, the point is that miracles and majesty are around us all the time. The question is not if they are there, but if we see them.

When Dr. Krueger chooses to enter Sacred Encounters with motherless twins and parents of critically ill infants, she is not trying to show off or to be a martyr. Instead, she is seeking to follow her life's calling. She also shows an awareness of both the suffering and the miracles that, like God, are always present. She once told me that people often say to her, "How can you do that kind of work? I couldn't." She used to be offended by the comment since it sounded as if these people were saying to her, "I'm too sensitive to do your kind of work." Now she appreciates that perhaps they are praising her for her courage.

> *...human life has no meaning without love.*

She sees her work as a calling. Those who see their work in this way, or at least understand their work as something they were meant to do, are far

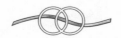

more likely to succeed in a Healing Hospital. That is where they can best express their work, in humility, as an "instrument of divine love."

THE HUMAN CRY

In the story of the housekeeper and the old man, the call of the old man for his daughter is a primal human cry that rises out of an agonizing admixture of physical pain and spiritual loneliness. It is a cry that rises from the throats of countless patients along the endless hallways of America's hospitals. It is a cry that, increasingly, either goes unanswered or is answered not with a loving hand but with a quick dose of medication from a busy nurse. The medication may put the patient to sleep, but it does not answer his or her fundamental cry for love. Is there anything more important? It turns out that after we have food and shelter, human life has no meaning without love.

Fortunately, there remain many caregivers who are still willing to offer love in the midst of chaotic work environments. These caregivers are entitled to the support of a loving culture.

ANOTHER SACRED ENCOUNTER: THE NURSE AND THE VERY TINY BABY

When I began working at Riverside Hospital in Toledo (now called Saint Ann), one of the most common causes of death was premature birth. In the 1970s it was difficult to save the lives of babies who were less than one-and-a-half pounds. At less than 500 grams, the situation was often hopeless. I remember talking with the staff in the special care nursery at Riverside Methodist in Columbus in the early 1980s. They would be caring for a tiny baby and I would ask them the chances for survival. They would often shake their heads mournfully.

Then things began to change. New treatments were discovered that made it easier to save the lives of these incredibly fragile beings. My visits to the neonatal nursery became more and more encouraging as nurse after nurse would give me a thumbs up when I would ask about the survival chances of their one- and two-pound patients.

Everything depends upon giving love unconditionally.

This was true, also, in the special care nursery at Baptist. Time after time, I would ask about the prognosis for a baby

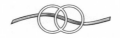

weighing less than two pounds, and they would astonish me with the news that the baby was doing fine. One evening, about 10 p.m., I stopped by the special care nursery in the course of making my rounds. I saw a nurse softly stroking the back of a very tiny baby. "What are his chances?" I asked enthusiastically. "Oh, this baby is dying," she said to my surprise. "He probably has less than an hour to live." I asked the whereabouts of the baby's parents and she told me they were too upset to be present. "This baby will die here with just me." A little while later the baby died right there in the full presence of that loving nurse.

What is so important about this story is that the nurse is not required by any law or policy to give this kind of loving care. At some hospitals she would be within the minimum standards of care if she simply checked the monitor of the dying baby until the heart rate line went flat. But this nurse believes in a higher standard. She believes in loving care. Radical Loving Care in a Healing Hospital calls *all* caregivers to the same commitment.

This nurse knew that the baby could not ask her to stroke his back in his final moments of life. She knew he would never thank her. Nevertheless, she gave her love completely and unconditionally, to a very tiny baby in his last moments of life.

This is what the Healing Hospital is all about. Everything depends upon giving love unconditionally. As Deschelle, a member of the house-keeping staff at Baptist said to me once, "Loving care means helping other people, no matter what!"

SACRED ENCOUNTERS IN THE GOLD ZONE

My object in living is to unite
My avocation and my vocation
As my two eyes make one in sight
Only where love and need are one
And the work is play for mortal stakes
Is the deed every really done
For heaven and the future's sakes.

— Robert Frost[28]

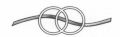

Today at Baptist is the last day on earth for two people and they are spending it in a hospital with their caregivers. It is the first day on earth for seventeen people, and they are spending it with another set of caregivers in another part of the hospital.

Birth and death are inherently sacred events — just as life itself is sacred. As caregivers, we can honor this sacredness. Unfortunately, many leaders and caregivers seem to have lost sight of the sacred nature of caregiving. The vise grip of the routine has strangled the meaning out of these exquisite moments. We all need help in reawakening ourselves to the joy of these labors. Almost every patient in-between life and death is experiencing some level of joy or pain — and all caregiving holds opportunities for Sacred Encounters. The joy in caregiving is as high as in childbirth and the pain may be as excruciating as an advanced cancer or death itself. Hospitals are places of extremes. That is why people come to them — for help in dealing with the extremes that have penetrated their lives.

No one comes to a hospital for entertainment. No one says on Saturday night, "What shall we do for fun? Hey, I know, let's check into the hospital!" The suggestion would be ludicrous. Hospitals are places of sacred occurrences. The problem is that many of the people who work there, deadened by the loss of passion for their work and mistreated by the system, have forgotten this. It is part of the goal of this work to reawaken this passion for the sacred work of caregiving.

We really need to try to get in touch with our own experiences of pain. I think of times when I have been nauseated from motion sickness or from bad food or from the effects of the Crohn's Disease that I have had since I was nineteen. I remember many nights lying alone on the floor doubled up with the painful spasms of this illness. Each of us has had times of suffering in our lives. The experience of pain is not only uncomfortable, it's terribly lonely. What is the medical treatment for loneliness? Pain has attached to it an anesthetizing sequel — amnesia. We are often unable to easily remember the depth of physical pain we have experienced. But we may remember the loneliness when we seek to reach out to a friend who is suffering.

It turns out that loving care is especially meaningful at times of either acute or chronic illness. One voice within us shouts, "Tough it out." Another part of us is scared and wants to be comforted. We want our mothers or our fathers, yet, as adults, we can no longer turn to them in the same way. This is the time when the warm and caring presence of a motherly or fatherly caregiver is a true healing presence.

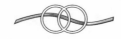

This highlights our original sacred encounter in human life. It is the earliest speechless encounter between mother and child. This is about our mothers not only feeding our hunger but also providing the warmth of their breasts, the stroke of their hands, and the soothing hum of their voices.

We have no conscious memory of these times of being loved as newborns, but every psychologist knows how critical it is that we receive this comfort. And every pediatrician and neonatologist knows that if newborn babies do not receive loving care in addition to food, they will typically lose weight and may die.

The concept of the Sacred Encounter arises in part from a sense of our relationship with God and in part from an understanding of the early comfort we received from the mother/father figures in our life. The importance of these early encounters demonstrates why we need the same thing later in life when we are sick. Adults, particularly men, may pretend that they don't really need love anymore, that it's "unnecessary." Yet for whom does a wounded soldier often call out in the midst of his agony? He screams for his mother. And whom do we yearn for ourselves in the midst of our greatest pains?

I vividly recall an experience with my own father with whom I was very close. He was a particularly "masculine" fellow — what we would today refer to as an "alpha male." My late father headed up YMCAs around the country for his entire career, and he kept himself in terrific physical condition. But in 1979, at age 74, he learned he needed bypass surgery. The night before the procedure, at the end of visiting hours, we all bid him goodnight and he smiled confidently at us. As we left and were walking down the hallway, I realized I had forgotten something. When I walked back into his room, he was sitting up in bed crying. There is no drug for this loneliness and fear but loving kindness and compassion. I reached out to him as best I could, but I was his son, not his mother or father. I felt very inadequate, and I thought about how we are never too old to need loving care.

The concept of the Sacred Encounter is simultaneously very simple and highly complex. At the simple level, a Sacred Encounter occurs whenever we meet another's deep need with a loving response. Our response may be intuitive, but love always assumes authentic intention.

At the same time, the Sacred Encounter is highly complex because we have begun to think of our relationships with others in such self-serving ways. It is extremely difficult to replace self-serving goals with other-serv-

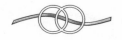

ing objectives. And the layers of painful need that a patient may have may be so complex that the patient may not understand them or be able to describe them. In other words, there is a deep need the patient feels, but he or she can't seem to describe it to us and therefore we have to make guesses. I reached out to my father with the particular love that children can give to parents. This met one level of his need, but there are so many other levels that I could not touch. If I had been more in touch with his need and my own ability to love, I would have dropped my self-consciousness and simply spent the night with him in his room.

A frontline caregiver may only need to understand the Sacred Encounter concept at the simplest level. Yet a deeper appreciation of complex patient need can significantly enhance the abilities of both caregivers and leaders in enriching the Sacred Work in the Gold Zone.

Sacred Encounters in the Gold Zone

Ordinary Work

Patient Need
"I need a glass of water & I'm scared."

Gray Zone

Transactional Response
"Here is a glass of water."

Sacred Work

Patient Need
"I need a glass of water & I'm scared."

Sacred Encounter Gold Zone

Loving Reponse
"Here is a glass of water. How may I ease your fear?"

The contrast to the Sacred Encounter is the day-to-day transactional encounter in which we interact purely for personal gain — to accomplish a particular job, to buy something or sell something else, to complete a task. These encounters are also essential to our lives, but each relationship can be dramatically enhanced by the concept of *authentic intention.*

In the first model above, it is always possible for us to stay bogged down in purely transactional encounters. When someone asks for a thing (*e.g.,* a glass of water) and also expresses an emotion (*e.g.,* fear) we can give them the thing and ignore the emotion. This excessive focus on task performance

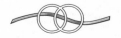

is the sort of thing that leads to demoralized staff members and unhappy patients. When a caregiver responds to emotional need with a transactional response, he or she has missed the opportunity to give love that could be healing, falsely assuming that patients "don't need that kind of stuff."

Transaction-focused caregivers are the ones most likely to end up burned out, not so much from fatigue as from loss of meaning. After all, transaction-focused caregivers often see their work as a function similar to that of an assembly line worker. With this view comes the attendant exhaustion and low self-esteem that such a self-concept generates. If I take care of gall bladders, my work is not very meaningful. If I take care of *people* with gall bladder disease, my work has endless meaning because my spirit can be engaged.

All leaders must understand how critical it is that the quality of work life be improved. Perhaps the world's most eloquent writing on this subject is from David Whyte. His books and poetry describe with great power the challenge that people face in seeking to open their hearts to their work. Whyte offers this encouragement:

> With a little more care, a little more courage, and, above all,
> a little more soul, our lives can be so easily discovered and
> celebrated in work, and not, as now, squandered and lost in
> its shadow.[29]

Whyte is painfully accurate when he writes about how this opportunity for the celebration of work is being squandered each and every day in thousands of work settings across America. Hospitals are among the worst offenders. Since the work is grim, we who work in hospitals often fall into the terrible habit of taking ourselves as seriously as our work. We want to think of our work as sacred or meaningful but find it difficult. If I am a patient transporter or a dishwasher, how can my work be meaningful? Of course, these people would need to consult the housekeeper in our story or to consider the example of Jesus when he knelt down to wash the feet of his disciples. It also helps if the leaders and co-workers around us, in times of both joy and sorrow, nourish our spirits. It is the responsibility of hospital CEOs to lead this celebration. Dr. Sallie McFague describes how critical the life of the spirit is when she writes:

> Life in the spirit is the only place where human beings can
> live fulfilled lives . . . God is not an 'extra' added on to life,

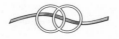

but life itself . . . Life takes place in love and for love . . .
When we become aware of God . . . as the source and goal
of everything and of all life, love, and power, then we
become channels for these realities.[30]

So the Sacred Encounter is the merging of "love and need" as Frost
writes (page 56). And to be powerful, this merging must truly be "for
mortal stakes." It requires the full commitment of a caregiver to meet deep
need. But it is also important to note that Sacred Encounters are not
limited to cases of dramatic pain. People in all kinds of jobs have the opportunity for Sacred Encounters of a different kind.

LOIS POWERS' POWER

A meaningful view of work as love's expression will often come from the
mouth or from the example of certain special partners in a Healing
Hospital, regardless of where they work. It is exemplified in a discussion I
had with a cafeteria cashier at Baptist named Lois Powers. When we say
that every partner in a Healing Hospital is a caregiver, how could this be
true of a person whose job assignment is to collect money and make change
each day in the checkout line? Lois found a way to love this work in a fashion that helped all those around her. I noticed the effect she was having on
people when I stood behind her one day and watched how everyone who
passed her would break into a smile or a laugh. She would often tell jokes
or touch people's arms gently as they went by her. Yet her line moved just
as fast as any other cashier's. The key to her success can be understood in
the way she describes her work: "I don't think of myself as a cashier, I think
of myself as a partner who has a special opportunity to brighten the lives of
other people. If a hundred people go by my cash register at lunchtime,
that's a hundred people I have the chance to make smile or feel better with
a little joke or a soft touch on the arm."

Lois changed the mental model of being a cashier. She redefined her job
in the way that every successful person does. Success often comes from
breaking out of the standard job description assigned to us. Why live inside
the tight prison of a written description? The best partners are always
thinking in the way Lois did. Needless to say, she was extremely popular
with all the employee partners. Equally important, she loved her many
years at Baptist Hospital. She brought her heart to work and was rewarded
with a long and satisfying career as a caregiver who happened to be

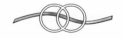

stationed at a cash register. This is an area where, certainly, many people could not conceive of the work as meaningful. Lois proved them wrong by her understanding of the second meaning of her work. She took the opportunity for hundreds of Sacred Encounters each day, and in her own way, managed to enter the gold zone during interactions that would often last only a few seconds. Again, Lois did not take any more time per encounter than other cashiers. Often her line even moved faster!

What we don't know, but can easily speculate, is the degree to which Lois's loving-kindness brightened someone's day at a deeper level. Her motherly love toward complete strangers may well have met the deeper need of someone who was feeling particularly sad and lonely as they passed her in the cafeteria line — and provided a moment of healing beyond Lois's knowing. It is clear that most visitors to the hospital have multiple encounters, so the effect is certainly cumulative — and powerful beyond anything Lois, or any of us, could know. Kind gestures always have ripple effects. So do unkind ones.

LIKE ONE BEING

Then I was standing on the highest mountain of them all, and round about beneath me was the whole hoop of the world . . . I was seeing in a sacred manner the shapes of all things in the spirit, and the shape of all shapes as they must live together like one being. And I saw that the sacred hoop of my people was one of many hoops that made one circle, wide as daylight and as starlight, and in the center grew one mighty flowering tree to shelter all the children of one mother and one father. And I saw that it was holy.[31]

— Black Elk

If we can think of ourselves as one people "like one being" as Black Elk says, then we can think of each other as brothers and sisters. This is, of course, also the teaching of Jesus. We are all children of God. We are all brothers and sisters.

This means that the man in tattered clothes who walks into the emergency department for the third time in a month bleeding and smelling of alcohol is our brother. It trivializes this person to refer to this kind of patient, as I have heard some ER staff do, as "the frequent flyer." The four-hundred-pound woman struggling in her wheelchair is not "the fat woman," but our sister. The unconscious drug addict, the angry old man on the stretcher, and the complaining country club socialite are all our

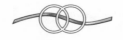

brothers and sisters. And each encounter holds the potential for the sacred.

When we take this view, then love may not seem so hard and kindness may come more naturally. In the most positive sense, our hospital policies must focus on giving the right medications rather than on not giving the wrong ones. Yet the clear warning in most hospitals is that mistakes will get you fired. As every high school basketball coach knows, a negative mindset most likely *increases* errors rather than decreasing them. We need to learn from this and start teaching positive thoughts rather than breeding negative ones.

For example, the way to motivate nurses to give the right medication is not to threaten them with termination for mistakes. This focuses energy and attention on errors instead of good nursing. Instead, they need to be taught that the reason to give the right medications is that it is an essential part of loving care. When meetings with patients are seen as potential Sacred Encounters, then the best care will naturally result.

Ultimately, the Sacred Encounter is a concept that can transform all of America's hospitals. Caregivers who have already been engaged in this kind of work may see opportunities for more of the same. Caregivers who have been stuck in a more transactional mindset may find themselves freed now to enter into work that holds real meaning. As they do this kind of sacred work, they may be startled to find that their burnout has "burned out." In its place is a new flame that glows within like a newly lighted candle.

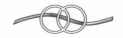

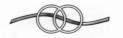

Chapter 5

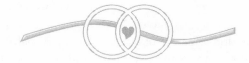

THE SERVANT'S HEART

It seems to me that now I learned at last what it means to love people
And why love is worn down by loneliness, pity, and anger.
— from "Meditation" by Czeslaw Milosz[31]

WHO CREATES SACRED ENCOUNTERS?

People who have a Servant's Heart create Sacred Encounters. Who are these people? These are people like the housekeeper who briefly stops her work to hold the hand of a sick old man and the special care nurse who spends half an hour stroking the back of a dying infant and the doctor who takes time in the middle of the night to comfort parents who are not even her patients. They are nurses like Deadre Hall, who prepares herself every morning by asking God to bless her only so that she can be a blessing to others, and Lorraine Eaton, who, instead of staying home on the lovely farm on which she lives, heads off to the hospital each workday to care for patients in a Medical Intensive Care Unit. These are people who understand, like Milosz, how "love is worn down." They know the need to refresh themselves with rest and meditation to support them in holding their balance as caregivers.

How do we identify and hire these people, and what kind of culture helps us retain these special individuals in our midst? The practical elements of these issues are discussed at greater length in Part Two. Here we will simply explore and learn to appreciate the nature of these individuals.

An individual who is primarily committed to serving others above him- or herself characterizes the Servant's Heart. Each of us has a Servant's Heart somewhere within, but it is pretty deeply buried in many. We start our experience of life thinking only of our own needs. As babies, we are totally dependent on our mother's milk and our mother's love. Our mothers, in fact, exemplify the loving behavior that meets the needs of a dependent baby. A loving mother is always thinking first about the needs of her baby.

We need to learn how to think like loving mothers when we are considering the needs of patients. We need to think about their needs above our own. Ultimately, it is some miraculous combination of both male and female energy that creates the ideal model of the Servant's Heart. This is what Martin Luther King called being simultaneously "tough-minded and tenderhearted." The Servant's Heart is expressed in the person who will offer kindness and caring but who will simultaneously be vigorous, even fierce, in the protection and advancement of a patient's needs.

The core image of the Good Samaritan is a sterling example. The Samaritan demonstrates courage in stopping to help someone in need who is of a different background. He chooses to stop when all others have ignored the injured person. He takes extra steps to ensure that the victim is cared for after he must leave him for a time, and he comes back to check on the victim later on in his journey. All of these actions are the choices of a person with a Servant's Heart.

We may not consider the actions of the Good Samaritan to be particularly heroic. The Samaritan did not do his work on the world stage with television cameras tracking his every step. He did his work quietly and unobtrusively and did not seek thanks. He gave his love unconditionally.

The housekeeper in her care of the old man replicates the actions of the Good Samaritan. We too can act with a Servant's Heart, and we too can be Good Samaritans in our work each day. To do loving work, however, we should not have to contend with supervisors who would punish us if we step outside our strict job description to help a person in immediate need. Every person in a Healing Hospital is a caregiver, regardless of his or her specific job description.

Clearly, there needs to be a process in place to ensure that a Healing Hospital is filled with people who have a Servant's Heart. This requires more than just hiring wisely. The Human Resources department cannot be

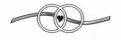

successful in hiring servants if orientation is so boring it puts these people to sleep and the supervisors on the floor are focused purely on efficiency. The entire system must support the actions of radical loving care. This means that hiring must be behavior-based, orientation must be inspirational and fun as well as informational, and review processes must reinforce loving care. It also means that employee partners who are unable to support this goal through their own actions must be respectfully removed from the organization.

The ultimate test of the radical loving approach is present in the consistent application of the Golden Rule. We must always ask ourselves: "How would we like to be treated if we were patients?" and "How would we like our mothers or our brothers or our spouses or our children to be treated if they were patients?"

It is important to attack again the notion that patients are just strangers. Once we have classified any unfamiliar person as a stranger, this may trigger a whole cascade of other images. Strangers are not friends. Strangers are to be feared. Strangers are people we should not reach out to because they may take something from us. Strangers are people with whom we shouldn't talk.

The mental image of strangers as people outside our circle of love is devastating to the concept of Radical Loving Care. Strangers must be incorporated in a new mental model built from the simple guiding principles that we are all children of God. Henceforth, patients are our brothers or sisters. This means that the homeless man who enters the Emergency department bleeding is my brother, and I will treat him not as a stranger, but as a brother to whom I will give loving care. The same is true for the five-hundred-pound woman struggling in her wheelchair. She is my sister.

The Good Samaritan did not ask whether the injured man by the side of the road was a stranger or not. He simply considered whether this was a human being in need of help. We cannot dismiss that incident by saying that times were safer back then — we can assume that helping a stranger was just as risky in the 1st century as it is in the 21st.

Isn't it wonderful to know that there are so many around us who have the potential to live out their work with a Servant's Heart? It is the challenge of a Healing Hospital to ensure that these special people are hired, oriented, trained, and retained in an environment where Radical Loving Care is the norm, not the exception. This is the challenge that every leader in a Healing Hospital must accept. It is the challenge of hiring the people who will be caring for our brothers and sisters in need.

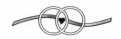

A HEALING APPLICATION OF COGNITIVE THERAPY

Leaders need to love their staff. I use the word *love* very intentionally here and ask you to reflect on it. Love doesn't require that we like each person but that we reach past liking to loving. We can adapt the work of Dr. Aaron Beck[33] in cognitive therapy to help us in this area. Cognitive therapy posits that our feelings and actions are influenced by our thoughts about a circumstance (or person), not by the circumstance itself. With simple yet powerful cognitive therapy, we can change our feelings and actions by rethinking our thoughts about others.

For example, perhaps I am a nurse manager who feels irritation toward one of my nurses when I see her yawn repeatedly during morning report. I discover that I am starting to dislike this nurse — perhaps I am telling myself that she is yawning because she is bored or is a disrespectful person. Taking a cognitive therapeutic approach, I can invite love to instruct me on how I can think about this situation. I hope the first thing my love would tell me is to give this nurse the benefit of the doubt. Perhaps she was kept awake all night long by a screaming baby or some other personal problem. Exploring other automatic thoughts may help me to change the distortion in my thinking (such as taking her actions personally, or "reading her mind"). Now I have a new mental picture of this nurse and the circumstance of her yawning. Through the lens of love I am forgiving and, incidentally, am likely to be a more effective leader for this nurse and her partners.

In over a quarter-century of hospital leadership, I have rarely heard managers talk about the love they had for their staff members. On the other hand, I often heard partners talk about how much they loved their team members. In American leadership, we generally have a false idea about the attitude the so-called "boss" is supposed to have for so-called subordinates. Of course, if the leadership model is control-oriented, love will probably sound like a strange notion. But love is exactly the attitude the Healing Hospital contemplates. The way to nurture people with a Servant's Heart is to model exactly the behavior we are seeking to advance.

The great team leaders I have known are passionately dedicated to their partners. They will make great sacrifices on their behalf and will routinely go far out of their way to offer help. This does not mean they are unwilling to be firm. The tough-minded/tenderhearted concept is as relevant here as it is for any aspect of the Healing Hospital. Demonstration of love by leaders toward staff is one of the best ways to break an old mental model and create a new and far better one.

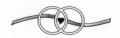

Chapter 6

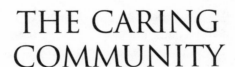

THE CARING COMMUNITY

We must convert our hospitals into caring communities.
— Keith Hagan, M.D.

THE FAMILY CARE MOBILE

Imagine a mobile. Each dangling piece is balanced delicately but powerfully in midair. Touch one piece and every other piece must move.

Now think of a family or a whole employee group like this. When one member is wounded, it affects all the other members. The laws of physics dictate that a mobile will always seek to right itself — to regain balance. A wounded family or a wounded organization will struggle to regain balance as well. This concept can help staff understand the need to be kind to family members as well as to the patient. In a Healing Hospital, family must not be shoved out of the caring circle but included whenever possible.

We introduced the Mobile Concept at Riverside Methodist Hospital in the early 1980s. We put the image everywhere to reinforce the significance of the idea. We hung a large mobile from the center of the lobby, and we even had a couple of images of mobiles etched into the glass of some first-

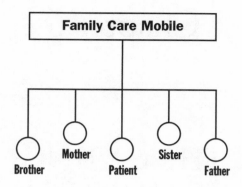

floor windows. This helped reinforce to our staff the many ways in which we are all connected. It reinforced, for example, the idea that when one member of a family has cancer, in a way the whole family has cancer. When someone close to us is sick, we too are affected. The mobile is jarred. To help both leaders and frontline staff members think like this is a good organizational application of cognitive therapy. The picture of the family mobile replaces our old idea that the patient is an isolated being and that nurses and doctors are his only caregivers.

As Marian Hamm, M.S.N., the wonderful former head of patient care services at Riverside, wrote to me one day, "There never has been a good day in a hospital. Someone is always dying and someone is always in pain." This means that the family mobile is being jarred all the time, and we must be attentive to the ways in which it can be balanced.

Although the patient may be at the center, everyone is affected by the severe illness of one, and the family should not be shunned. In less-developed countries, this culture of caring is actually more developed, and whole families may move into a hospital to help care for a loved one. Such a practice need not be seen in America's high-tech centers when sterile fields may be critical, but at the same time, family members should not be straight-armed simply to honor an overly strict rule. An obvious example is that visiting hours don't really have to end precisely at 8:30 p.m. when the patient is dying of cancer. The family can be an enormous help in the care of a patient.

In addition, as Moore and Komras emphasize in *Patient-Focused Healing*,[34] "probably the most significant determinant of success or failure

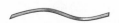

in patient education is the patient's family, including friends who serve in a support role." And yet for decades now, the family members have been needlessly marginalized by a system that emphasizes rapid discharge of the patient. This approach is counter to healing because it fails to recognize that patients discharged from acute-care settings are undergoing a startling transition from complex technical and skilled support to home settings that have neither. The Healing Hospital approach, therefore, emphasizes the active engagement of the family as much as possible. This involvement also furthers healing by reducing the chance that the patient will have to be readmitted because of errors made by family members in supporting the patient at home.

In the same way, a team of caregivers can become a family unto themselves governed by the concept of the mobile. In a Healing Hospital, employee partners feel their connection to every member of the team. When one member is ill or having performance problems, every member of the team (every piece of the mobile) will be affected. Like the mobile, the team will attempt to balance itself. In a hostile environment, the rest of the team may shun a weakened team member. In an environment of radical loving care, balance occurs as each member seeks to support and help the one who is out of balance.

CARE CIRCLES, CARE PARTNERS, AND CULTURE SHIFT

Radical loving care cannot be accomplished without creating a culture of loving service. It is the culture of loving service out of which radical loving care arises. A series of small systems creates the caring community that is the guiding force of such a culture.

The worst kinds of bureaucracies are characterized by platoons of people who have been reduced to robots. In broken bureaucracies, human beings perform functions that may seem completely meaningless to them. As a result, they feel their work is meaningless and therefore they must be meaningless. This can lead to cruel behavior by bureaucrats. A leader in this kind of bureaucracy may become a "little Hitler" wielding abusive power over subordinates in a raw attempt to infuse himself with power and a sense of meaning. After all, the culture suggests that nobody cares anyway, since no one is really a human being. Since efficiency is the alleged God of the bureaucracy, why should anyone care about a human being's true need?

The caring community of a Healing Hospital works to defeat abusive

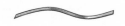

leaders and meaningless environments. Two small but powerful tools can support leaders in accomplishing a culture shift from meaningless bureaucracy to caring community. The first is a Care Circle. Briefly, the Circles are groups of ten or twelve employees (called partners) who meet periodically to give partners the opportunity to share concerns with each other. In these meetings, each partner takes five minutes to share with the group how things are going in their lives and any concerns they wish to raise with the group. Each other member of the group listens respectfully and supportively. Our work with this model demonstrates that it is one of the best single ways to build a sense of commitment and community around mission.

The second program is called Care Partners. Care Partners are a committed group of employees who are assigned to care for all patients aged sixty-five and older. These partners are not patient advocates. The patient advocates concept is well intended, but the title suggests that a patient advocate is an adversary to the rest of the staff. Instead, Care Partners act as stand-in family members and are supported by Care Companions. The first head of the Care Partner program at Baptist is Perri Lynn White. Under her direction, Care Partners work to ease the concerns of older patients by being present to them — either in person or by phone — twenty-four hours a day. Although Perri Lynn remains as head of this program, the initiative has, unfortunately, been cut back at Baptist Hospital on the grounds that it is too expensive. This is unfortunate, as it is likely that the program saves more than it costs in terms of reduced patient falls, reduced calls by the patients to other caregivers, and increased overall patient satisfaction.

Both of these programs are described in more detail in Part Two. What is critical in this chapter is to understand the fundamental concept. Radical Loving Care requires, and will generate, changes in the tired old systems that have been choking out love for the last several decades. The new systems will free employee partners to do their best work in environments where they are affirmed as people of dignity and worth. They in turn will treat patients and each other the same way. This is the essence of a caring community.

Caring Cultures: Key Summary Points

1. The guiding image is a caring community, not a bureaucracy.

2. Relationship and efficiency are both important.

3. A caring community operates as a partnership in which staff work with each other (partners), not for each other (employees).

4. Simple guiding principles are more important than rules.

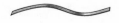

Chapter 7

THE LAYERS OF MEANING IN RADICAL LOVING CARE

It is not how much we do, but how much love we put into doing it. It is not how much we give, but how much love we put into giving.

— Mother Teresa

From now on in America, any definition of a successful life must include serving others.

— George W. Bush

lthough it should seem obvious, it is unfortunately necessary to state that people do not metamorphose into one-dimensional beings when they become patients. Quite the contrary, our emotional needs increase when our bodies are weakened. We need to look to the multiple meanings a patient presents to us.

PRESENCE AND POWER OF MULTIPLE MEANINGS

One way we can understand loving care is to create a model of the whole person that schematically portrays two core elements of our totality (see diagram below). Just remember that if we think too mechanistically, along the lines of the Cartesian model which bifurcates mind and body, we run the risk of categorizing human needs as mental *or* physical. This division has plagued medicine for the past two centuries and seems to increase in severity with each passing decade. The model below should not be interpreted as a way to reinforce this division but as a way to deconstruct a human model of wholeness with the assumption that our thinking will be led to reconstruction along a more enlightened pathway.

The Layers of Meaning in Radical Loving Care

Total Loving Care = A Higher Standard

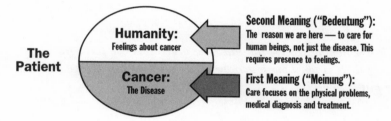

The Patient

Humanity: Feelings about cancer

Cancer: The Disease

Second Meaning ("Bedeutung"): The reason we are here — to care for human beings, not just the disease. This requires presence to feelings.

First Meaning ("Meinung"): Care focuses on the physical problems, medical diagnosis and treatment.

In the German language, the word "meaning" has two meanings. The philosopher Hans Gadamer, through the use of the words *Meinung* and *Bedeutung*, emphasizes the fascinating split in the nature of these terms.[35] Meinung, here, refers to literal meaning. When a leg is broken, this "means" that it needs to be fixed. It also means a certain number of weeks in a cast, using crutches, and so forth. Bedeutung implies a larger or *second* meaning. In the case of a broken leg, the Bedeutung is the larger significance of this event in the life of the patient. What will it do to the patient's life to have a broken leg? How does the patient *feel* about the fact that his leg is broken?

Our spiritual life, of course, encompasses both First Meaning (Meinung) and Second Meaning (Bedeutung). The word spirituality is often attended by religious overtones. Here, spirituality is to be thought of in the broadest possible way. Our spirituality is both our "otherness" as well

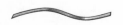

as our wholeness. It is the mystical, soulful aspect of humans that transcends body and mind. As my wife has said to me, "Our bodies are but the temporary homes of our spirits," and they need to be honored as clay touched by God.

How are caregivers expected to approach this quality in a patient? The Healing Hospital approach encourages a *ministry of presence* to the patient as a spiritual being. My colleague, Perri Lynn White, who heads the Care Partner program at Baptist, told me she likes to think of the passage from Hebrews in this context: "Do not neglect to show hospitality to strangers, for by doing that some have entertained angels without knowing it."[36] Nancy West, executive director of Nashville's Siloam Clinic, which serves the poor, says, "We like to think of each patient as the face of Christ." These models of thinking are enormously helpful in generating respect by caregivers toward patients. They also serve to elevate the role of the caregiver. Once I think of you as a spiritual being, I am more likely to be able to respond to you in a loving and balanced way. Simultaneously, I am less likely to think of you as merely a broken machine in need of repair. This kind of thinking also elevates the nature of my work — I care for the children of God, not for derelicts or foreigners or drug addicts.

> *Once a person has been reduced to "the gall bladder," it is easier to leave her sitting alone in the hallway...*

The body-as-machine model is what causes caregivers to think of patients as "gall bladders," "diabetics," "broken legs," or some other disembodied part of a human being. This objectification of people is what causes dehumanized and unloving treatment. Once a person has been reduced to "the gall bladder," it is easier to leave him sitting alone in the hallway outside the Radiology department. After all, it's not a person who's been kept waiting, it's just (subconsciously, of course) a gall bladder. Consider the effect of this language on caregivers. If I am only taking care of gall bladders, I'm sort of a body mechanic. If I am caring for children of God, my work is truly spiritual.

THE NEED FOR "SECOND MEANING" CARE

The Second Meaning, or Bedeutung, does not appear on an X-Ray or MRI, of course, but it is of vital importance. This second meaning must be the special focus of our loving care. It is not a mechanistic expression of the person. Therefore, it must be perceived not by our literal nature, but by our

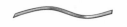

second nature. We can only perceive the needs of second meaning in the same way we see nature itself — by slowing down, by pausing, by listening with our hearts as well as our minds.

Our spiritual life represents a unity of these two levels of meaning. It goes beyond and within both meanings to suggest an even deeper element of the spirit. This impossible-to-define element remains intact regardless of what has happened to the body or even how the patient might feel emotionally or think analytically. Again, the way to address this spiritual meaning is to acknowledge it by being present to the needs of the person before us.

Much of this thinking on spirituality is, by nature, highly intuitive and can be as challenging to a concrete thinker as working on an assembly line may be to an intuitive thinker. One is not necessarily more important than the other. The key point is that each of the two meanings must be thought of in the context of the other.

In the typical hospital, a patient's expression of spiritual need brings calls for the chaplain. In a Healing Hospital, *each* caregiver must be trained and supported to honor the emotional needs of patients. This does not necessarily require *more* time from caregivers but, instead, suggests that the time of the caregiver be spent in a different way.

Interestingly, loving care does not require twice the time, but it does require more than twice the *presence*. Caregivers in a Healing Hospital cannot enter a patient's room looking hurried or rushed. They must always have a sense of presence to the patient.

The Golden Thread of mission and vision calls us to remember that we are part of a beautiful and meaningful tradition. It calls us to honor our heritage of loving care as long as it is within our grasp. It also calls us to never lay it down, but to be an example for those who come after us — and to hand the thread to them as they take on the responsibility to be loving caregivers.

PLACEBOS *VS.* MEANING

The so-called "placebo effect" is a classic illustration of the impact of loving care. In a brilliant article on this subject[37] brought to my attention by Roy Elam, M.D., Drs. Daniel Moerman and Wayne Jones attack the use of the word "placebo" as inadequate and inaccurate to the degree the word "placebo" is used to minimize the impact of psychosocial forces. They believe that the placebo effect should be renamed the "Meaning Effect"

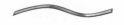

because it so clearly and powerfully affects the physical healing of patients as well as their emotional state.

They cite several studies demonstrating the phenomena of patients reporting improvement when they have been given an inert substance instead of an active drug. They even cite the example of surgery on mammary arteries as a treatment for angina. "Patients receiving sham surgery did as well — with 80% of patients substantially improving — as those receiving the active procedure..."[38]

We can draw a powerful conclusion from this and other irrefutable evidence. There is a whole range of things that doctors and nurses do with patients that have a big impact, including things that have *nothing to do with direct medical treatment*. These things include the effect of the white coat the doctor is wearing[39] (it raises blood pressure in some patients) and can logically include the tone of the doctor's voice or the demeanor of the nurse.

Consider how you feel when someone enters the room. We all have a particular response to any change in our immediate environment. Sometimes we may be unaware of it, but when we think about it, we can see how we are affected. For example, if the person entering the room is a stranger carrying a gun aimed at us, our heart rate and blood pressure will obviously go up quickly as we experience the fight or flight response. On the other hand, if the person carrying the gun is a trusted friend of ours playing a joke, our reaction will be different. What if the person is carrying nothing at all but is someone we see as an enemy? What if it's a friend who's a great comedian and brightens the room for us just by his or her entrance?

All these dynamics apply to the entrance of any caregiver into our room. The irritable nurse who enters the room with a scowl on her face is not likely to promote healing. The caregiver who comes in with warmth and kindness can surely help us on our way to recovery.

All of this suggests that in a Healing Hospital, staff members need to be trained to be attentive to the power of the Meaning Effect. Imagine the impact on nurses who begin to appreciate that their manner in entering a room can be therapeutic for the patient — or not.

Ultimately, the passion here is to be *com*passionate to others, freely and openly. Caregivers need to allow their kind natures to be their regular way of being. Surely this is what God, and each patient, wishes from us in our caregiving.

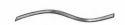

THE HEALING CARE FORMULA

Because caregivers work in a science-biased environment that often grounds decision-making in formulas, it may be helpful to visualize how Loving Care fits with Clinical Care in a formulaic model (see diagram). The components being added together may seem like apples and oranges — yet they make up the essential fruit of the caregiver's life.

Healing Care Formula

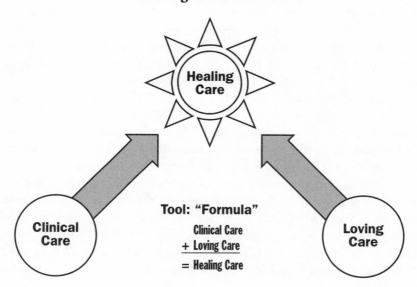

Note that just as clinical excellence does not guarantee a cure, the healing formula does not guarantee healing. In fact, one of the important understandings about healing is the notion that *a person may be physically healthy but not healed, while another person may not be physically cured, yet may be healed.*

Can a person recover physical health without love? Perhaps we can partly answer this question by asking another: Can a person sometimes recover physical health without medical treatment? The answer to both of these questions is, of course, yes.

The need for loving care is highlighted by recalling, again, the discussion I had with the orthopedic surgeon, who said that if a patient came to him with a compound, comminuted fracture of the right leg, it didn't

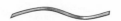

matter to that leg whether it got loving care or not. The leg, he said, would get better based on the skill of the surgeon in successfully treating it. What I said was, "You may be right. The leg doesn't need loving care to recover. But the leg is attached to a person, and the person *does* need loving care."

> *...what is likely to be more healing: a love-based encounter or a transaction-based encounter?*

Ultimately, however, the more important question in a Healing Hospital is not *can* a person recover without love, but what is likely to be more healing: a love-based encounter or a transaction-based encounter? Some combination of the two is integral to effective care in a Healing Hospital.

And there is always the "Mother Test." What would *you* prefer for your mother: to have her cared for as a gall bladder or a breast cancer, or to be cared for with loving clinical excellence, as a human being?

NECESSITY AND SUFFICIENCY IN HEALING CARE: A HIGHER STANDARD

We all know that loving care is not required by either the law or by the Joint Commission on Accreditation of Healthcare Organizations. No hospital or doctor can be successfully sued on the grounds that they did not love enough. In the Healing Hospital, we do not deliver loving care because law requires it, but because it is the right thing to do. It is a higher standard of care that Healing Hospitals set for themselves.

An organization that seeks to be healing needs to post a version of the Healing Care Formula everywhere. More important, the formula must be posted in the mind and the heart of each caregiver.

The truth, here, is that every person who seeks to serve with a Servant's Heart wishes to open his heart to the expression of love. As Rilke wrote, "I want to free what waits within me / so that what no one has dared to wish for / may for once spring clear / without my contriving."[40]

The partner with a Servant's Heart will consistently break free of self-interest and do the utmost for any patient at any time. These servants understand the role of physical care as *necessary* but not *sufficient* for the full care of a patient. In other words, for a severely broken leg to be healed, it is necessary that the leg be set. The setting of the leg is necessary, but the setting of the leg alone is not sufficient to meet the standard of a Healing Hospital. For this standard to be met, the physical care given to the patient

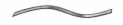

must be expressed in a loving fashion. This may require that we pay attention to the effect a broken leg has on the emotional state of the patient. For example, does it cause him or her to feel depressed because of the temporary life limitations imposed by the injury? How can we help the patient deal with those feelings?

Several years ago I saw an exquisite example of a doctor practicing empathy when I went on rounds at the University of Wisconsin hospital with my brother-in-law, Dr. Stuart Updike, a nephrologist. Stu was caring for a teenage patient with diabetes. The previous day, he had prescribed for the patient a new wearable device to enable the easier and more effective delivery of insulin. The device required that the young patient have a subcutaneous needle placed in his stomach. As Dr. Updike examined the needle placement, he asked how the patient was doing with the new device. The patient looked a little uncertain, whereupon Dr. Updike lifted up his shirt to show that he was wearing the same device himself and had the same kind of needle inserted in his stomach! He had simply replaced insulin with a neutral solution. The pleasantly surprised teenager beamed at the doctor and said he was doing just fine. A physician willing to align this closely with his patients is clearly a caregiver with a Servant's Heart.

PATIENTS AS PEOPLE IN LIMINAL STATES

One of the essential ways to come to a better understanding of the need for love in the Healing Care formula is to consider the concept of *liminality*. As my colleague and editor, David Cox, has explained it to me, "Liminality has to do with the experience of transitioning from one space to another. One is in a liminal phase when one is no longer in the old state but not yet in the new state."

Interesting examples of this have to do with rituals of passage. Anyone who has parented a teenager, or just plain remembers being one, recalls the awkwardness, the "liminality," of this state. Adolescents have neither the freedom of childhood nor the confidence of adulthood. They are in transition. The same is true of immigrants as they transition from their old familiar world into a new one.

David tells me that Vanderbilt Divinity School Professor Howard Harrod, who died of cancer, spoke eloquently about how living with terminal cancer was like living in a perpetual liminal state. You are never "cured," but neither are you dead — and people treat you as if you are somehow different from other people, from healthy people.

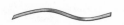

Beyond this, Professor Harrod's immersion in the liminal state was rein-forced by his own sense of alienation following multiple surgeries in his genital area:

> . . . I gradually became aware of how deep my gender social-ization had been. Not only had I a sense of having been mutilated, I had also lost the very capacities that were sym-bolically associated with manhood in American society. I no longer had a prostate, I was incapable of an erection, and I had no testicles. More fundamentally, I had lost the capacity to experience desire . . . surrounded by the presence of youthful Eros . . . I began to feel a crushing weight of loss.[41]

But Dr. Harrod subsequently discovered that, in a strange way, he gained something as well. He was able to express love for his wife with a complete absence of sexual desire. There is a remarkable inference we can draw from this. Since sexual desire arises as an appetite, then we may con-clude that desire itself is an appetite. Our personal appetites, the Siren's songs that appeal to our physical needs, may be a root cause of much of our unloving behavior toward others. Theoretically, it would be easier for us to be loving caregivers if we had no strong physical needs of our own. And yet it is the presence of these personal needs of ours that makes love's expression so powerful. It is our willingness to put aside our own needs in favor of the needs of others that is often seen as the sacrifice called for by loving care.

We may draw a key distinction between desire and passion and think of desire as a physical need that can never fully be satisfied, while passion is spiritually driven and may as such be fulfilled. When loving care is a mas-querade coming from an insincere caregiver whose motive is simply to earn a paycheck or a promotion, than the energy source is desire and the behav-ior will ultimately lead to a burned-out employee. On the other hand, when loving care comes from the authentic expression of a passionate care-giver, it is not only powerful, but it is fulfilling. This authentic passion is what I see in the hearts of caregivers who clearly love their work — whether they've been doing it for three months or thirty years.

Of course it needs to be understood that no human being is perfect and even the most passionate of caregivers has moments of fatigue and weak-ness when the competing demands of the body are overwhelming. This simply reinforces the need for all of us to 1) take good care of ourselves and

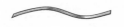

allow time for self-healing and 2) cut each other some slack so that when otherwise committed caregivers have a bad day, we can forgive them and they can forgive themselves.

Meanwhile, the attack of disease experienced by a patient is often followed by a second attack — from the surgeon. Parts of us are cut away and we begin to wonder what parts of us are essential to our identity and our humanity. In the midst of all this, we not only find others looking at us differently, but we look at ourselves differently as well. This sense of being changed leaves us feeling intensely and acutely vulnerable. Caregivers can ease these feelings or unwittingly reinforce them depending on the degree of their loving presence.

A dear colleague of mine, Rhonda Swanson, told me about the alienation she felt in the midst of her cancer treatment. In spite of people's best intentions, one is treated differently, like a person banished from the arrogant fraternity of the healthy. Rhonda felt this especially when she lost her hair. After wearing a wig for a while — a specific effort to cross the bridge from liminality back to the land of the healthy — she finally abandoned it. "The wig isn't me. This is who I am," she told me, indicating her chemotherapy-shortened hair, "whether my hair is long or short or not even there."

Human existence in the liminal state cries out, in particular, for loving care to be combined with clinical care, as the Healing Care Formula prescribes. Joining the two together is the only way to achieve true clinical excellence.

THE MYSTERY OF PAIN AND SUFFERING

As a beginning trial attorney, I was familiar with the legal concept of pain and suffering as it relates to damages in a civil trial. A plaintiff asks for multiple kinds of compensation from a defendant. First she or he asks for damages for the "actual" injury. For example, in an injury case in which the plaintiff has suffered paraplegia, "actual damages" refer to things like out-of-pocket medical expenses for care. In addition, it is common for attorneys to demand compensation for the pain and suffering their client has endured.

How are juries supposed to calculate the dollar value of the suffering that a paralyzed person endures? The client's legs may have lost the sensation of pain, but there is no end to his or her suffering. Nevertheless, typically, the American legal system charges juries to calculate monetary

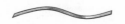

damages for both pain and suffering when liability has been determined. Our society consistently applies metrics to the essentially immeasurable because we respect the importance of things like pain and suffering even though they cannot be calculated with precision or X-rayed like a broken leg. So to further the ends of justice, complex and indescribable pain and suffering is converted to hard cash.

It is essential that every caregiver who seeks to be part of the continuous chain of love in a Healing Hospital have the best possible appreciation of and respect for the pain and suffering of both patients and family members, to remain constantly sensitive to the fact that pain that cannot be measured is nevertheless deeply real to the patient. But caregivers who were perhaps compassionate early in their careers may find that their hearts have become hardened by years of inadequate support and appreciation from leaders.

Further compounding this problem is that many of us have a certain amount of amnesia about our own pain experiences. We often avoid thinking about the hardest suffering we have experienced, and we may have anesthetized ourselves from current pain by using drugs or alcohol. Practices that enhance the understanding of pain can include visualization exercises that help caregivers remember pain they have personally endured. This can help us understand the significance of presence to those who are enduring pain at this moment.

Included among those worthy of compassion are an important group of patients that are sometimes ignored unintentionally. These are the patients who are unconscious, those we think can stand certain pain because, "after all, they won't remember it." It's remarkable that we justify both inflicting and ignoring pain merely because it will later be forgotten. Does this mean we can operate on patients with Alzheimer's without an anesthetic or otherwise cause them pain just because they will forget it? Few would agree that such a practice should be tolerated, and yet we do essentially the same thing with some infants and with unconscious people. Until very recently, male babies subjected to circumcision were not given any anesthetic. Thankfully, most hospitals have finally changed this practice. I have seen beautiful examples of compassionate caregivers in recovery rooms and intensive care units who consistently treat unconscious patients with exquisite kindness. I have also seen unconscious patients subjected to various levels of abuse by caregivers who apparently thought they were doing no real harm. Unconscious patients need to be treated with compassion and respect as if they were conscious.

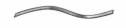

At the same time, we all understand that pain is often a part of the recovery and rehabilitation process. The key is to use the principle of respect to guide our actions. It is the responsibility of all healthcare leaders and doctors to ensure that strong guiding principles are in place to assure the respectful treatment of unconscious patients and babies.

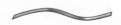

Chapter 8

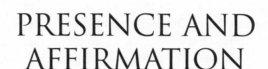

PRESENCE AND AFFIRMATION

Those who do not run away from our pains but touch them with compassion bring healing and new strength . . . wanting to alleviate pain without sharing it is like wanting to save a child from a burning house without the risk of being hurt.[42]

— Henri Nouwen

It requires courage to show up for life — to be truly present to each other. Many of us used to be present, but it got too painful. We are always running the risk of being hurt in the course of our caregiving as we may have been elsewhere in life. Back when we were kids, we showed up for Christmas until we found out there was no Santa Claus. After that, if we showed up, we may have appeared with a certain guarded reserve — a reluctance to really appear because we might again be tricked.

The reason it is so important for caregivers to establish real presence with patients is that it's the only way to truly appreciate the patient's needs. This presence is especially dramatic with patients who have altered consciousness. This includes patients on respirators with tubes down their throats who struggle to speak their needs and cannot. How can we learn their needs?

One of the heartbreaking realities of a technology-driven hospital culture is that it becomes too easy to turn our backs on patients who can't speak. In the film *The Servant's Heart*, the caregivers demonstrate exquisite sensitivity to the needs of their patients. This is because they imagine themselves into the patient's misery. Instead of turning away, they stay with a patient until they can feel enough of that patient's pain to truly understand the need. As manager Debi Villines, R.N., says, "We can't turn away from a patient's pain just because it's difficult."

Is this difficult work? Of course it is. Is it worth doing? Yes, if we are truly interested in meeting the needs of others. If we truly care about people, we will work to change how we care for people. In almost every case, serious illness or injury has more than an effect on the part of us that is machine-like. D.H. Lawrence wrote powerfully about this at the beginning of his poem "Healing":

> *I am not a mechanism, an assembly of various sections.*
> *And it is not because the mechanism is working wrongly, that I am ill.*
> *I am ill because of wounds to the soul, to the deep emotional self...*

Lawrence speaks further of the need for time and patience in the healing process. Time and patience are the gifts of a caregiver with an ability to be present. In this time, in our world of high velocity and complex demands, many caregivers may need to relearn the meaning of presence. In *Waiting for God*,[43] Simone Weil wrote, "The capacity to give one's attention to a sufferer is a very rare and difficult thing; it is almost a miracle; it is a miracle." It is painful to share the pain of another. In addition, David Whyte has pointed out that the velocity of our daily life includes stunning demands for our attention from thousands of directions simultaneously.

> *The most basic and powerful way to connect to another person is to listen. Just listen. Perhaps the most important thing we ever give each other is our attention.... A loving silence often has far more power to heal and to connect than the most well-intentioned words.*
> — Rachel Remen, M.D.

Henri Nouwen has written eloquently: "It is of the greatest importance that we leave the world of measurements behind when we speak about the life of the Spirit." This is very difficult for medically trained people to do. For some, the worthlessness of measurement in this context is best understood when we ask ourselves the question, "How much do we love our children, or our mothers, or anyone else we love?"

Antoine de Saint Exupery addressed this issue when he wrote in his remarkable book *The Little Prince*, "It is only with the heart that one can see rightly. What is essential is invisible to the eye." In order to be present to the needs of the heart and the spirit, we need to let go of calibrations and calculations and simply seek to be present to need.

Simple presence may not feel like enough, yet it is a precious gift currently withheld (unintentionally) from most patients. It is a gift that lives within all good caregivers. Leaders need to develop "presence training" for all staff.

What does it mean to offer this training? George MacDonald wrote that in order for us to truly come alive in this world, "we must wake our souls unnumbered times a day." We all need training to refresh us and to keep our souls "ajar," as Emily Dickinson invited us to do, "always ready for the ecstatic experience."

Leaders must begin by learning what presence is all about. Clearly, it requires setting aside time to dedicate to this work. Make no mistake, the notion of real presence has become an important new discipline, and its effective expression has become one of the keys to creation of a Healing Hospital. Good psychologists and leadership trainers are typically aware of what it means.

As Thomas Merton points out: "Those who do not run away from our pains but touch them with compassion bring healing and new strength . . . " How do we stay near in the midst of someone else's pain? Alternatively, how do we avoid reducing our reaction to pain to a simple transaction in which we administer drugs but never engage at a human level? There is no avoiding the call of love, to be present to another's need, and to remember that "to alleviate pain without sharing it is like wanting to save a child from a burning house without the risk of being hurt."

TRACY'S PRESENCE AND MICHELLE'S AFFIRMATION MAGIC

Healthcare in America seems to have lost its way . . .
— Tracy Wimberly, R.N.

When Ms. Wimberly speaks these words, she is referring in part to the way healthcare has slipped off the path of balance and has gotten lost in the woods of money and technology. Tracy is the person who has taught me

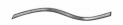

the most about the power of healing presence. She is my long-time colleague and dear friend, and she devoted her entire rich career to helping improve the quality of life for caregivers. Early in her healthcare career, Tracy understood the meaning of presence and how it could affect the healing of patients. Across her distinguished life of work, first as a public health nurse, then as a nurse educator, and then as a senior executive responsible for everything from patient care to human resources to the design of environments, she campaigned ceaselessly to create settings that would affirm the people who lived, worked, suffered, and celebrated in hospitals.

It was Tracy who taught me that the notion of healing presence is critical to the success of a Healing Hospital. It's like the presence of a parent to a child. If our child wants us to listen to her or him, what signal does it send if we are watching television at the same time? Clearly, the child will not feel valued. The same is true of adults. It is particularly true of those sick adults known as patients.

*Healing presence...
is what makes a
patient encounter
sacred.*

Full presence to patients signals they are valued. Split presence signals they have less worth and value. A robotic presence that treats the patient encounter as a transaction signals to the patients that *they* are robots.

Healing presence changes everything. Healing presence allows both the patient and caregiver to experience the sacredness of their encounter. Called or not called, God is present. And this is possible even for the nurse who feels he or she has no time. I have seen harried nurses engaging in these kinds of encounters many times. They understand that presence can be signaled in seconds. It does not require hours of handholding. It is the gift that comes from a Servant's Heart. It is also a skill that can be developed as long as it begins with *authentic intention*.

It's important for each of us to think of individuals in our lives who demonstrate the marvelous skill of being truly present to us. One of the most magical people I have ever met in this respect was Michelle Jackson. Michelle and I were students together at Vanderbilt Divinity School, and Michelle was a part-time chaplain at Baptist Hospital. Tragically, Michelle, who was afflicted with a chronic lung disease, passed away suddenly, in June of 2003, at the young age of thirty-eight. She had just received her Master of Divinity degree from Vanderbilt. The flood of notes following her passing, and the rich texture of those notes, reflected Michelle's remarkable gift of presence.

Person after person described Michelle as one of the most luminous people they had ever known. Her radiant smile and endless brown eyes always seemed welcoming and never passed judgment. Love flowed through her freely and unconditionally. It has been said that it's not that important what we say or do but how we make other people feel that counts most. Michelle made me feel accepted.

It may be relevant to note that Michelle was a young African-American woman who loved casual clothes while I am a middle-aged European-American male who often feels required to wear business suits. Of course she didn't care about any of that. She would just come up and give me an enormous smile and a huge hug — a hug so great that any sense of superficial difference between the two of us would fall away. It seemed to me that every encounter with Michelle was a sacred one because her presence was always so complete. For this to occur, she had to offer her unique kindness *and* I had to be willing to receive it — which was extremely easy with Michelle.

Literally hundreds, maybe thousands, of people felt about Michelle the same way I did. How did she do this? Ultimately, it was not about what she *did*, but who she was. She was a loving person. She listened to what was special about each person she met, and she always seemed to remember it. If your father had died, she would remember that and ask you about it in subsequent meetings, and when she asked, it would be as if she cared as deeply as if she had known him — because she *did* care.

As a hospital chaplain and as a friend, Michelle provided as good an example of presence as I ever encountered. She did not believe she was a perfect servant, but, to me, she was a perfect friend. Through the transparent skin of her soul, people could gaze into a mirror and see their better angels. In this sense, she was a healing presence to anyone open to her gift. You may know someone with a gift like Michelle. If you do, you understand what I mean by the healing power of presence, and how important it is that we cultivate this gift in caregiving.

Once each of us has made the core decision that other people are our brothers and sisters, a radiance starts to shine through us. It is the radiance of God's light. Beyond my inadequate words, I hope you can see that light from Michelle. It is the light you may see in anyone who has the great strength to give you the best gift life has to offer — unconditional love.

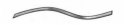

PRESENCE AND POETRY

After Great Pain

After great pain, a formal feeling comes
The Nerves sit ceremonious, like Tombs
The stiff Heart questions was it He, that bore,
And Yesterday, or Centuries before?

The Feet, mechanical, go round
Of Ground, or Air, or Ought
A Wooden way
Regardless grown,
A Quartz contentment, like a stone—

This is the Hour of Lead
Remembered, if outlived,
As Freezing persons, recollect the Snow
First Chill then Stupor then the letting go

— Emily Dickinson

This indescribably powerful description of the aftermath of pain tells us so much about pain and the power of poetry in helping us understand it. Reading and writing poetry, or music, or attempting any art is about making an effort to understand and describe the invisible things. These things seem to come more within our reach after we have struggled to describe them — and had the courage to stay present with them — instead of bolting and running for the false comfort of some safer ground.

What is the feeling after great pain? It can be the formal and noble sensation that comes when we discover that pain has finally released its grip and we have won the struggle for now. The body relaxes a moment and the mind takes a breath. Poetry and the other arts are, like pain and joy, hard to touch and to hold. When William Blake writes, "He who kisses joy as it flies by/ lives in eternity's sunrise," he reminds us we cannot hold joy in a box. Pain is often hard to remember as well because we *don't* want to hold it.

It's hard to persist with poetry because it can be so painful, as may be

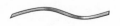

evidenced by the suicides of poets Anne Sexton and Sylvia Plath. It can be equally painful to stay close to music, as Mozart and Beethoven both found, and we know the tragedies of other artists like Van Gogh and Gaugin. Magnificent art is a great fire that can cast light and warmth and can also scorch those who come too close.

Still, staying open to art can teach us at a deep level about compassion and presence — and it can help us overcome our amnesia about pain so that we may better understand the agony of others. When we open to art, we are increasing our ability to see and hear and, most of all, to feel. That is why presence to art can teach us about presence to the needs of others among us who are in pain.

There is another reason for us to engage art in our lives every day. It is because the noise of the rest of life constantly conspires against the loving side of us. The day's demands tend to capture us in a vortex of velocity. This may keep us busy doing so many different *things* that we have trouble experiencing any *one* thing. We jump from one task to the other, devoid of the kind of reflection that is critical to a life of presence as a caregiver. I described this once when I was trying to express the elusive chance for joy in one of my days:

Crimes of Omission

A day like this is rich with music.
You may think every day has music
and you would be right. Yet, often
I cannot hear the day's songs. The noise
of phones will not make room. Every morning
the chatter of the day clatters against the dawn
and drives away the soft moon. And the cavalry of my lists
shoulders aside memory and Mozart and Liszt.

A day like this has roses in it.
You may think every day holds roses
and you would be right. Yet, often
I cannot see them. Their wet petals

and intimate fragrance are concealed from me
by the whir of conditioned air and electric screens

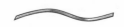

and dead white pages that rise
like ghosts to dim my hours. And my quick hands are so busy

with busy work they fail to slow a moment to brush
the skin of a single rose with my fingers
or hold a solitary note of music in my palms,
or embrace you on a day
that holds each of us in its arms.

Poetry helps us take a conscious breath and inside that breath to hear and see and touch — and feel something we would not have felt had we not paused. Like miracles, like love, and like God, poetry is there if we will just notice it. Poetry, and all the arts, lives at the intersection where we encounter the common thread that binds all of us together in both joy and pain. It is here where a nurse can convert what might have been a typical surgery or an ordinary birth into a sacred experience for patient and family — and her. She does this with the quality of her presence. Multicolored threads turn gold at the intersection of poetry and love, pain and joy, and birth and death. It is up to us to see this gold and celebrate it, for it is here where mind and heart weave together to form the rich tapestry of our spiritual life. This tapestry is always there, waiting for us to discover it.

Richard Moss wrote, "The greatest gift you can give another is the purity of your attention." Those who have been able to find quiet in the midst of this raucous world so that they can give their purest attention to the voice of God are the ones who create great poetry and music and art and literature. We may follow their example and, in so doing, create great caregiving through our presence to the world of the ill. This gift of presence is something each caregiver can cultivate.

Chapter 9

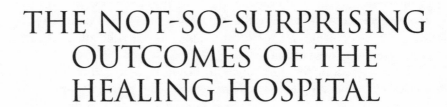

THE NOT-SO-SURPRISING OUTCOMES OF THE HEALING HOSPITAL

Come, my friends, 'tis not too late to seek a newer world.

— Tennyson

DOING THE RIGHT THING

The best reason to build a Healing Hospital is that it is the right thing to do. Our mission statements all say that we believe in caring, and the Healing Hospital is about balancing loving care with traditional clinical care, so it is quite clear that the only thing to do is to restore this balance.

In order to accomplish effective cultural change, employee partners need to be treated for who they are — whole persons, not just functionaries. The same concepts that transform care of patients apply with equal force to employee partners. It is heartbreaking to contemplate the degree to which so many employees are denigrated in their work. In talks with leaders around the country, I have heard frontline staff members referred to as "the little people," "the lower-level staff," and even "the units of expense." Staff members referred to like this are not likely to receive much loving leadership.

Sadly, these examples and the logic in the first paragraph above are not powerful enough to solve the problem. In a transactional world, the simple fact that holistic leadership is the right way to lead is not enough to motivate most organizations. Two other motivators remain: 1) the motivation of *outcomes* and 2) showing *how* to create such a place. There is a need to demonstrate a clear method of building a model that can deliver this kind of loving care.

Fortunately, a few pioneering organizations have already restored love to the center of care. For example, the best news about the story of the housekeeper and the old man is that the story is true. It is held up as a positive example of loving care at Baptist Hospital in Nashville, the birthplace of the Healing Hospital concept.

It bears repeating that love should be placed at the center of the medical care model because *it is the right thing to do*. This reason is sufficient in and of itself. No other reason is really needed. Every mission statement in America talks about "caring." None of those statements say that the reason to care is that it brings a good return on our financial investment. But interestingly, doing the right thing typically generates measurable positive returns.

> *...doing the right thing... generates measurable positive returns.*

OUTCOMES OF DOING THE RIGHT THING

It may be a shock to many that the love-based model is not only the right thing to do, but is the most successful way to run a hospital from a quantitative as well as a qualitative standpoint. It may actually be dangerous to focus too heavily on the positive returns. They may be so appealing that they could be seen as the *only* reason to put a Healing Hospital Mission in place. But let's take a brief look . . .

In two large complex hospital systems in two different states, the essence of the Healing Hospital model has been applied with stunning results. In the OhioHealth System (that includes Riverside Methodist Hospital in Columbus), outcomes improved dramatically across a twelve-year period starting in 1983. Income rose from $2 million to $56 million, patient and employee satisfaction rose to the top percentiles, turnover in nursing sank into the single digits, and job applications to work at Riverside skyrocketed.[44]

Outcome measures in five areas at Baptist Hospital in Nashville are

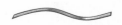

powerful indicators of the success of the Healing Hospital model. Although the Healing Hospital initiative was not formally named until January, 2001, the same basic approach was being used before the name was applied.

OUTCOMES AT ONE
HEALING HOSPITAL

1998-2001 AT BAPTIST NASHVILLE

The reason to build a Healing Hospital is that it is the right thing to do and has great outcomes:

1. **Patient Satisfaction.** In the last quarter of 1998, prior to the initiation of the Healing Hospital effort, inpatient satisfaction hovered around the 68th percentile (Press-Ganey system). After three years of work on changing the culture at Baptist, patient satisfaction had risen to the 99th percentile for hospitals of similar size and the 97th percentile in the category of all hospitals regardless of size.

2. **Employee Morale and Turnover.** In 1998, employee turnover hospital-wide was 29.4%. By June, 2002, turnover was down to 15%. Even more significantly, turnover among Registered Nurses had dropped from 24.7% to an impressive 8.5%.

3. **JCAHO.** In August 2002, the Joint Commission on Accreditation of Healthcare Organizations paid their once-every-three-years visit to Baptist. After an exhaustive (and exhausting) four-day survey, the Commission awarded their findings. The hospital was awarded a score of 98! This is the highest score in the hospital's history and among the highest awarded to large hospitals anywhere in the country. In addition, there were no Type 1 violations of JCAHO rules, which are the worst kinds of violations.

4. **Clinical Performance.** Though somewhat harder to measure, the perception at Baptist is that clinical performance has improved. Nurses are

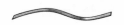

focused on giving the right medications every single time, not just on the negative of avoiding mistakes. Patient restraint policies and practices reflect the presence of loving care rather than forcible control. Problems are solved in *dialogue*, not by edict.

5. The Bottom Line. As mentioned in the first chapter, one week after I became President of Baptist, the hospital reported a bottom line loss of **73 million dollars** for the year prior to my arrival, fiscal year 1998. By fiscal year 2001, that loss had been significantly reversed and the hospital showed a gain of nearly one million dollars. The central strategy in this turnaround revolved around an incredibly simple model of concentric circles that was so helpful in providing a basis for change that everyone understood — even if they didn't agree with it. It placed the patient (P) at the center. Cost reductions were guided by the proximity of a person or an activity to the center.

The Rings of Care

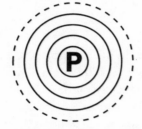

In the five-circle model, the first circle represents direct caregivers; the second, support staff; the third, middle management; the fourth, senior management; and the fifth, ancillary activities of the hospital, including ownership of real estate, sponsorship of professional sports teams, and ownership of physician practices.

The theory is that the farther an activity is from the center, the more important it is to reduce or eliminate it. Herein lies the reason most leaders fail to adopt a model like this — it puts them in the fourth ring out from direct patient care! Yet by following this model rigorously, we were able to create savings, energy, *and* commitment together with a new and powerful belief that we would succeed — which we did!

When the hospital system was finally sold, it was sold at a fair price to new owners, Saint Thomas Health Services. We felt confident they 1) would carry on and advance our loving mission, and 2) had the financial stability to ensure the long-term operation of the organization.

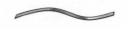

PART TWO

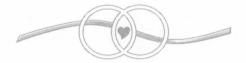

The Blueprint
For a Healing
Hospital

The Development of Radical Loving Care

*Every truth passes through three stages before it is recognized.
In the first, it is ridiculed. In the second, it is opposed. In the
third, it is regarded as self-evident.*

— Arthur Schopenhauer

Breakage

I go down to the edge of the sea.

How everything shines in the morning light!

The cusp of the whelk,

the broken cupboard of the clam,

the opened, blue mussels,

moon snails, pale pink and barnacle scarred—

and nothing at all whole or shut, but tattered, split,

dropped by the gulls onto the gray rocks and all the
     moisture gone.

It's like a schoolhouse

of little words,

thousands of words.

First you figure out what each one means by itself,

the jingle, the periwinkle, the scallop full of
     moonlight.

Then you begin, slowly, to read the whole story.

— Mary Oliver (2003)

Chapter 1

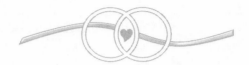

LAYING THE
FOUNDATION

Our deepest fear is not that we are inadequate, our deepest fear is that we are powerful beyond measure. It is our light, not our darkness, that most frightens us. We ask ourselves, "Who am I to be brilliant, gorgeous, talented and fabulous?" Actually, who are you not to be? You are a child of God. Your playing small does not serve the world. There is nothing enlightened about shrinking so that other people won't feel insecure around you. We were born to make manifest the glory of God that is within us. It is not just some of us. It is everyone. And as we let our own light shine we unconsciously give other people permission to do the same. As we are liberated from our own fear, our presence automatically liberates others.

— Nelson Mandela[45]

LEADERSHIP COMMITMENT

I recently surveyed a group of over one hundred leaders at a major hospital. I asked them a range of questions about a Healing Hospital and what it took to create one. The vast majority of them indicated that without CEO support the initiative would be dead in the water.

They may be right. It is clearly possible to initiate many of the Healing

Hospital ideas in parts of the hospital, and the ideas described here about loving care are things any individual caregiver can practice every day, but the whole-hospital initiation of this work is difficult to advance without deep leadership support.

Most of us are, unfortunately, inclined to play small. But leaders cannot take this luxury. They need to find courage and advance this work, remembering Mandela's enlightened observation that "as we are liberated from our own fear, our presence automatically liberates others."

Fortunately, a growing number of hospitals are deciding to initiate this work or to add it to their existing strategic plans. When you think about it, why would you want to run a hospital any other way? The Healing Hospital concept represents everything good that can happen in healthcare. It is the kind of organization of which we would all like to be a part. It is the kind of place we would want our families to come to as patients. It is the kind of place that our communities deserve.

Still, these ideas can be difficult for some CEOs to buy into because they require a fundamental rethinking of the CEO's job and a deep recommitment to the core of mission. It's a lot easier to just ignore the challenge and stay in the comfortable status quo. And even a CEO who is open to change is likely to want someone else to be the pioneer and take the initial arrows.

I invite you to be part of this pioneering effort. As President Mandela says so well, "Your playing small does not serve the world." It is time for American healthcare leaders to be part of the most important change in the history of healthcare leadership. As we "let our own light shine we unconsciously give other people permission to do the same. As we are liberated from our own fear, our presence automatically liberates others." This is the kind of leadership that will make a genuine difference in the lives of countless caregivers and their patients. This is about leaders trying to do the best for their staff and patients. It's about being able to say, at the end of each day, that we're part of something truly meaningful — the work of giving loving care.

THE BOARD

Most boards spend a stunning amount of time hearing financial reports, listening to plans for new buildings or the renovation of old ones, evaluating business plans, or reviewing the minutes of previous meetings in which they did the same thing. Clearly, all of these activities have their

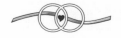

place. But where is the agenda item that focuses on the actual human care of patients? Where is the report from the CEO on what he or she is doing to support the morale and energy of frontline staff members?

In a Healing Hospital, the Golden Thread of loving care weaves its way through the entire agenda. This means that clinical, business, and care issues are all discussed in the context of what is truly best for patients and staff. As obvious as this sounds, I have rarely seen this approach practiced in a sincere way. Instead, board committee discussions can quickly degenerate into competitive language about beating the hospital across town, or meaningless discussions of how to beat down some third-party payer, or how to get the edge on a vendor. These kinds of discussions do not serve the interests of either staff or patients.

Board support is critical to the creation of a Healing Hospital. For the positive reasons mentioned above, giving support should not be hard to do. What board would want to say no to a leader who wants to create a loving, healing environment in line with the mission statement of the organization?

The Baptist Hospital Board, under the capable direction of Virgil Moore, offered me all the support I needed. In addition, Mr. Moore and the board have continued to support the Baptist Healing Hospital mission right through the merger and into our new organization, The Baptist Healing Hospital Trust. This kind of support is absolutely crucial in the advancement of a loving mission.

Most hospital board members are, by nature, somewhat conservative. This means they may resist change, even when the change is clearly for the good of the organization, and even when the change involves simply living out the existing mission. There is always the risk that a given board will get cold feet and decide to retreat to the status quo. This is why it is so critical that leaders step forward to advance the loving care agenda by insisting that the board hear regular reports on what the staff is doing to advance loving care.

An enlightened board with strong leadership will naturally embrace the mission and vision of a Healing Hospital. On careful analysis, it will be seen to be the only true and wise way to lead a hospital organization. This approach works particularly well with board members who are given the opportunity, through a retreat, to understand at a deeper level what a Healing Hospital is about.

A Healing Hospital is the natural outgrowth of any good mission and vision statement. If the mission statement is something like, "We are a

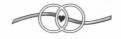

caring organization devoted to providing the best clinical care to the community in a cost-effective way," then the Healing Hospital approach is perfect. If the organization simply wants to puff up the bottom line, there's no need to waste time in the sacred work of a Healing Hospital.

Board members need to be given the opportunity to understand and embrace the loving care approach. For example, it is helpful for them to know that loving care is *more* than just kindness. Loving care calls for exceptional stewardship of resources. It calls for high performance in clinical areas. And it calls for a renewed commitment to honor the trust placed in a hospital by its community.

Most of all, the Healing Hospital approach calls for renewed dedication to the creation of a continuous Golden Thread of loving service. This thread weaves unbroken through every caregiver and every executive and every doctor and every board member. The board is the governing body, and the adoption of the Healing Hospital model needs to be embraced by the board as a core philosophy.

MEDICAL STAFF

The great danger of the increasing professionalization of the different forms of healing is that they become ways of exercising power instead of offering service.

— Henri Nouwen[44]

It can be a harder task to gain the support of the medical staff. We have had limited success with that at Baptist Hospital. This is not because doctors have actively opposed the effort — it's because, frankly, we haven't tried hard enough. The process needs a dedicated leader who will devote significant time to it. At Baptist, we have had the great gift of the leadership of Dr. Keith Hagan, who continues as chairman of our Program Committee at the Trust. Still, he is a practicing physician whose main role is to care for his own patients.

Most doctors already believe they're engaged in giving loving care and this may well be true. But I have also encountered many doctors who just don't think of loving care as being very important in the treatment of illness. Does this surprise you? If you are one of those who think everyone in a hospital believes in the criticality of loving care, I will recall for you the conversation I had with the orthopedic surgeon. In more detail, it went something like this:

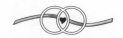

Doctor: "Erie, this loving care stuff is nice, but frankly, if I have a patient with a compound, comminuted fracture in his right leg, that leg is going to get better by skilled treatment, not because I give it loving care."

Erie: "Maybe the leg doesn't need loving care. But the leg is attached to a person. And that person does need loving care."

Doctor: "Well, maybe."

This conversation encapsulates the challenge of advancing an intuitive model around loving care in the presence of people who think more concretely. It also reinforces why D.H. Lawrence felt the need to say, in his poem quoted earlier in chapter 8 in Part One, "I am not a mechanism, an assembly of various sections." And caregivers must never again be confused by the notion that because human beings have machine-like parts they can be treated like machines.

In any case, my suggestion is to go ahead and build the culture among the employees first and draw selected physicians into the movement along the way. It's not that there will be great physician opposition. The problem is generating enthusiasm for something that seems "soft" to many. There *will* be sympathetic physicians, and energy should be focused there. Where attention goes, energy flows. So it's good to stay with the positive. If a single strong physician emerges as an advocate, as Dr. Keith Hagan did at Baptist, this is tremendously helpful. A group of physician advocates can be built from this, and after that a significant percentage of the medical staff can be brought on board.

As every hospital leader knows, doctors are deeply upset and discouraged by the current healthcare environment. Actually, this is an understatement. So many doctors are upset that there has been a sharp decline in medical school enrollment and a concurrent rise in early physician retirement.

Thousands of physicians joined together recently to demand fundamental change in the healthcare reimbursement system by calling for a single-payer government insurance program. As the authors of an article in the *Journal of the American Medical Association* wrote recently, "Physicians and hospitals would be freed from the concomitant burdens and expenses of paperwork created by having to deal with multiple insurers with different rules, often designed to avoid payment."[47]

This is the kind of environment in which we are offering the concept

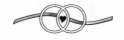

of the Healing Hospital. It is actually an appeal to the better angels within every doctor. It is a call to the best reason to become a doctor in the first place — to heal the sick because they are sick, not to become bogged down in questions about the patient's payment system. I believe this is what all good doctors seek — the ability to practice medicine without undue interference. This is the core of the appeal of a Healing Hospital.

RESOURCE COMMITMENT

Financial priorities must be shifted to come into line under the simple guiding principle that mission must drive the bottom line, not the other way around. This means primarily signaling new support for caregivers consistent with the concentric rings of the care model described in Part One.

The good news here is that this whole effort should be able to be launched without significant resources because it relies on using existing staff. The only costs should focus on training and on the creation of teams of Care Partners and Care Companions. These programs will be discussed more fully in chapter 6.

TELLING YOUR STORY OF LOVING SERVICE

One of the most powerful ways to communicate the Healing Hospital Story is effective filming of frontline staff as they are engaged in the mission of loving service. World-class videographer Van Grafton and I have worked for several years to develop the skill to shoot and edit stories of caregivers at work into moving and effective films for presentation to healthcare audiences around the country. The two films we have completed to date are *Sacred Work* (2001) and *The Servant's Heart* (2003). If you want to see examples of powerful storytelling, I encourage you to acquire copies of these films through www.healinghospital.com. They are fantastic teaching tools and are more effective than anything else in describing the power of this work.

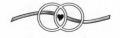

Chapter 2

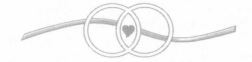

ILLUMINATING THE GOLDEN THREAD OF HEALING

From the point of view of Christian Spirituality, it is important to stress that every human being is called upon to be a healer.

— Henri Nouwen[48]

We have some nice people here and there.

— former president of a major teaching center referring to caregivers at his hospital

Once upon a time, several years ago, I interviewed the president of one of the largest and most prestigious hospitals in the world. At the end of the interview I asked him an odd question. I asked if he would choose his own world-renowned hospital if he needed to be a patient. He gave me a surprising answer. He said no. He said "I'd go to the BI [Beth Israel in Boston] because Mitch's people take such good care of you over there."

The "Mitch" he referred to was Dr. Mitch Rabkin, former president and CEO of Beth Israel Hospital in Boston. Dr. Rabkin and his team had so radically changed the culture of that hospital that, back in the '80s, many proud locals would often say, "The best hospital in the world is Massachusetts General, but the best hospital in Boston is Beth Israel!"

I asked the leader of that prestigious hospital why he would not want to be a patient in the place he ran. He said, "Our primary goal here is research; second comes teaching." He put patient care last on the list. When I asked him if he didn't have caring staff, he said, "Well, we have some nice people here and there."

Inside the last part of his answer is the center of a problem about loving care in hospitals. Every hospital has "some nice people here and there." The problem isn't the people.

The obstacle to continuous loving care rests in part with the leadership. With rare exceptions, leaders fail to support frontline staff in giving the loving care that is needed. I am confident this CEO did nothing to change care at that hospital after our meeting. After all, he knew that he could go to a different hospital if he needed to be hospitalized.

> *Sadly, most missions don't matter. Most vision statements don't count.*

In essence, that leader apparently failed to shape a vision that advanced patient caring at the bedside. By listing his goals in the order he did, he gave the stunning impression that it was impossible to have great research, teaching, and patient care all at the same time. Aren't research and teaching supposed to improve patient care? Yet as many leaders in university hospitals will admit, patient care often does come last.

From the 1970s up into the 1990s, Dr. Mitch Rabkin, a true leader with a Servant's Heart, created a mission that mattered and a vision that counted at Beth Israel Hospital. His leadership transformed the lives of both caregivers and their patients. Unfortunately, his successful commitment to patient care is rare in western medicine.

Tennyson says comfortingly through Ulysses, "Come, my friends, 'tis not too late to seek a newer world." And it is not too late for us to pursue a new vision. But the time to change the world of healthcare is certainly long overdue. It will continue to be difficult to reverse the ingrown wrongheaded patterns of the past several decades. Loving care is very hard work. Yet in healthcare, it is the only work worth doing. It means deep love. It means being kind to those who are rude and being loving when you're

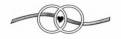

exhausted. It means constant concentration on giving the best quality of care and it means being honest in the face of criticism. This work can be exhausting. Yet if we look both into this world and beyond it, we will find that this work is what our lives are meant to be about. This work is our calling.

If we choose to accept this call of loving care, our work will take on deeper meaning because we will be making a bigger difference in the lives of others.

Many of those we choose to help will never thank us. Therefore, I would like to thank you for choosing to increase your commitment to living out your love for others. It may be the best choice you and I can ever make.

THE GREAT UNFINISHED BUSINESS OF HEALTHCARE

"Next Sunday we all went to church . . . The men took their guns along . . . It was pretty ornery preaching — all about brotherly love, and such-like tiresomeness; but everybody said it was a good sermon, and they all talked it over going home, and had such a powerful lot to say about faith, and good works, and free grace, and preforeordestination, and I don't know what all, that it did seem to me to be one of the roughest Sundays I had run across yet."
— Mark Twain, *Adventures of Huckleberry Finn*[49]

"Brotherly love," as Mark Twain says through the character of Huck Finn, really does sound like so much "tiresomeness" to many people. That's because it's eloquently preached but infrequently practiced. Instead of loving one another, we are encouraged to beat one another in sporting events, kill one another in wars, and to "get the edge" on one another in business.

Part of the thesis of this book is that the notion of seeing other people as rivals with whom we have self-serving transactions is a wrongheaded view that has infected the healthcare world like a contagion. Just like the "ornery preaching" that Huck Finn complains about, we talk endlessly in hospital mission statements about caring for the ill. In reality, hospital leaders focus most of their energy on the latest technology and the bottom line.

With special yet rare exceptions, the tentacles of technology, dragons of business, and dungeons of bureaucracy have driven loving care from America's hospital rooms and operating suites. The leaders and practitioners of American healthcare need to renew the ancient commitment to

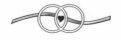

support the healing of the whole person. We need to put love at the center of this healing wheel. This wheel has many spokes that will be explored further. In order for this wheel to turn, every spoke must be in place and must be sturdy and strong.

In America's not-for-profit hospitals, the mission must drive the wheels of the business model, not the other way around. This focus on mission is both the legal basis for tax exemption and the ethical basis for the existence of not-for-profit hospitals. As one of healthcare's few great spiritual leaders, Dan Wilford, former President and CEO of the giant Memorial Hermann Healthcare System in Houston, has said, "Our ministry must decide our business plan, not the other way around."

The question in the Human Resources department must not be simply does this candidate have an educated mind, but does he or she have an educated heart. We must ask, does the candidate for a caregiver's job have what we call in a Healing Hospital a "Servant's Heart"? The question in the Capital Equipment committee must not simply be which department gets which piece of technology, but how that technology best serves our mission of total patient care.

In the midst of the pressures of daily work, can we, as leaders, step back for a moment and look at the larger picture of our mission? Are we being who we say we are, or are we falling into the hypocrisy that Mark Twain lampooned so often and so successfully? Are we following the hard discipline of ensuring that loving care is a continuous chain throughout the illness care experience? Are we supporting our frontline caregivers in this mission, or are we sending them signals that efficiency and the bottom line are all that matter?

All hospitals have a responsibility to place love at the center. Hospitals grounded in the Judeo-Christian tradition, in particular, are the last, best hope to restore loving care to the place Jesus intended it to be. In faith-based hospitals, we understand that we are all children of God and, therefore, we are all brothers and sisters. The Healing Hospital is grounded in these notions and offers a template for how to carry forward this sacred work in a series of Sacred Encounters.

It may not be time for a revolution, but it is time for a revelation — the discovery that the opportunity is before us today. It is time for us to act. If not us, who? If not now, when? If not here, where? If we, as leaders, are not guiding a hospital toward the goal of loving care, then where are we leading it?

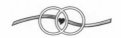

REVOLUTIONIZING MISSION AND VISION

Great minds have purposes; others have wishes.

— Washington Irving

Our hospitals' missions need to matter. They cannot be merely impossible-to-remember paragraphs framed on the wall. We need volcanic vision statements that explode the tired but persistent old patterns of mediocrity. Our staff and patients are depending on us, but they may not be expecting much. Many have grown skeptical. They've heard promises before and seen them abandoned.

We must lead our hospitals toward being what they say they are. Leaders have the opportunity to set the agenda. The mission of loving care will be the underpinning for every issue addressed by our hospitals. Our vision must come leaping off wall plaques and into our hearts and our hands. It must pervade every aspect of our work.

Sadly, most hospital missions don't matter because leaders never illuminate the Golden Thread of the organization. Missions hang on the wall gathering dust. Likewise, most vision statements don't count. For that matter, most books on leadership fail to improve anyone's leadership. Yet all mission statements are high-sounding. The problem is that most missions, visions, and leadership books fail to awaken the energy to live out the words on the wall or in the pages.

Our vision statements need to be engraved in our hearts, not just on plaques. It takes enormous energy to live out what we believe. It takes a deeply committed person to change a life pattern in favor of a better one. The challenge lies not in the intellectual acceptance of an idea, but in the living it out.

We all believe in truth, but do we tell it all the time? We all believe we should love one another, but do we practice it as much as we think we should? Motivating a hospital family to live out the principles of the Healing Hospital requires committed leadership. This is a challenge that most leaders have not yet accepted. As leaders we have let the Golden Thread fall from our hands. We have failed our frontline staff. We have not given them the support they need, and it is time for us to embrace a vision that will change all of that.

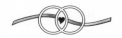

MISSIONS THAT MATTER AND VISIONS THAT WAKE US UP

That's what's wrong with the world. There's way too much reality happening.

— character in the movie *Still Breathing*[50]

Most missions melt in the fire of everyday "reality happening." It takes extraordinary leadership to combine a mission with a strong vision to bring about meaningful change. Mission and vision statements should call out to us. They should awaken our best instincts and help motivate us to live out the language of hope. But what have we done with most of our mission and vision statements? These are the statements that describe who we are and how we would like to live out our organizational lives. Generally we have posted these words on the wall in compliance with accreditation requirements, but we have failed to engrave the words in our hearts. Can you recite the mission or vision statements of the healthcare organization for which you work? Can people on the front lines do the same? What counts is that we live the words we hold up as our reason for being.

Our mission and vision statements must be bold! No one has ever been motivated by a vision that calls for small, incremental change. Can you imagine being inspired to follow a leader who stands before the management council saying, "Let's go out there and make some minor changes over time!" or, "Let's get out there and maintain the status quo!" Yet this is essentially the message that most leadership teams send to their staffs.

Effective mission and vision statements 1) are clear and easy to remember, 2) make a strong call for dramatic improvement in the lives of others, and 3) are announced by leaders who, through their example, demonstrate a passionate commitment to making them come alive.

For example, Jesus came with a radical new message of love. No doubt it shocked his listeners to hear Jesus say, in the Sermon on the Mount,[51] that although they had heard before that revenge was appropriate (an eye for an eye and a tooth for a tooth), now they should not only love their friends, but love their enemies as well.

Martin Luther King's dream was a bold call for the complete integration of the south. Imagine if he had said, "It would be a nice idea if black people and white people could get along a little better." Or what if his vision statement had simply been, "To improve race relations." From the standpoint of many white southerners in the 1950s, improving race rela-

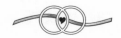

tions would simply have meant to keep things the same. Fortunately for succeeding generations, King insisted on a vision for radical change and created both the words and the actions to back it up.

In a different way, Herb Kelleher's vision for Southwest Airlines was another kind of radical change. Many scoffed at his notion that employees of an airline might actually have fun in their work. When Kelleher combined his vision for fun with a workforce of committed employees and an action plan focused on low-cost, reliable service, a uniform use of Boeing 737s, and a simple seating system, he revolutionized air travel. Astonishingly, even though passengers and airline experts have applauded the Southwest model, most other airlines have yet to follow suit.

What's particularly brilliant, and often underappreciated, about Kelleher's work is that he awakened his employees with a vision that they could have fun and joy in their work and also create a great airline! I have been interviewing Southwest employees for years and have yet to encounter one who doesn't love his or her job. At other airlines it is common for the first employee I meet to quickly complain.

As of this writing, Southwest is clearly the best-performing airline in the country in almost every category that counts — including profitability. The company's leadership is a prime example of living out King's message of being simultaneously tough-minded and tenderhearted.

When we read that Walt Disney articulated a vision of "the best in family entertainment," we can see in retrospect how much sense that makes. Disney could see it at the time. All we have to do is consider the worldwide impact that the Disney organization has had over a half-century and we can see the power of that vision and the creative and passionate example Disney himself set.

With the possible exception of the Mayo Clinic, hospital organizations are noteworthy for their conservatism and predictability. The notion of revolutionizing care has been largely limited to changes that are driven by technology or pharmaceuticals. Actual loving care has been left behind or shoved to the sidelines.

Hospital mission statements about caring have turned out to be mostly well-intentioned fabrications of high-sounding words that most people have no intention of living out. Consider the harried admitting clerk in the ER. When you come to her with a pain in your side, will she ask you about your pain, or will she instead demand your name, address, and insurance card? What about the underpaid patient transporter who comes to take you to your room? What about the temporary radiological technologist who

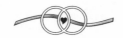

comes to photograph your insides or the nursing technician who comes to take your clothes?

> *Unfortunately, that job description is silent about the gift of love.*

Interestingly, each and every one of these people, when asked, will say they believe in loving care. Yet none of them gets much support from the system for living out that vision. Instead, they are given the message that they need to follow their job description. Unfortunately, that job description is silent about the gift of love. Why not paint the color of our love into our gray workday — each of us in his or her way?

At the beginning of this work, I described the crisis I found at Baptist Hospital when I arrived. It was not only a financial crisis but a cultural crisis as well — a crisis flowing from an unfortunate departure from mission. Mission and values are usually drawn up in the midst of sunny skies. In times of crisis in many organizations, the values are the first to go. Some leaders look for extra weight to throw overboard, and the finance people usually start to sharpen the chain-saws for a massive layoff. Notions about kindness, respect, and loving care may be quickly sacrificed on the altar of financial survival.

I share all of this to tell you that our leadership team at Baptist decided to do something unusual in the face of this trouble. In the midst of the organizational storm, we gathered our several thousand employees together in groups of about a hundred at a time. I asked all the staff the same question. What is the most important thing we do here?

Everybody knew the answer: It's taking care of patients, of course. In each meeting, after this answer was given, I drew a circle on an overhead slide with a "P" in the center for patient. Then I drew concentric circles out from the center to represent the rings of people who care for patients — starting first with the direct caregivers.

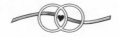

APPLYING THE RINGS OF CARE

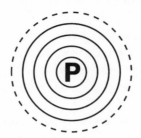

In the five-circle model first seen in Part 1, the first circle represents direct caregivers; the second, support staff; the third, middle management; the fourth, senior management; and the fifth, ancillary activities of the hospital, including ownership of real estate, sponsorship of professional sports teams, and ownership of physician practices. The farther an activity is from the center, the more important it is to reduce or eliminate it. The logical expression of this theory is that cuts should start at the outside and move in. This means that, as much as possible, the outer ring should be eliminated and the fourth and third rings should be reduced.

We secured the full support of the Board — especially the leadership of Virgil Moore, Willie Davis, Scott Jenkins, and Ken Ross. Dr. Bob Norman also did a lovely job of keeping us focused on our mission, and we had the gift of having Keith Hagan, M.D., as president of the Medical Staff.

Excess real estate was sold as fast as possible, and we sold one of our small hospitals. In addition, physician practices were aggressively disgorged from Hospital ownership. This moved hundreds of people off the payroll who did not actually lose their jobs, because most were able to continue as employees of the doctors who were now back in private practice.

We were unable to escape our sports sponsorship contracts, but the effort to do so helped maintain our credibility and proved that we were serious about cutting away things that were remote from patient care. Next, the top seven managers at Baptist, including me, took voluntary pay cuts during 1999. In addition, as President, I removed about one-third of the administrative staff.

At the same time we announced, at the end of 1998, that Baptist planned to hire one hundred more nurses! This kind of action can infuriate financial officers, but it thrills doctors, caregivers, and the public we serve. Ultimately, it brings other rewards.

These basic steps laid the foundation for a dramatic financial recovery.

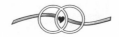

What I believe really saved Baptist Hospital from bankruptcy was the new spirit and renewed commitment of our leadership team and all 3500 of our employee partners.

But saving a hospital is about more than just saving its bottom line. For any of this to matter, it is necessary to convert the culture into a truly healing organization. Otherwise, who really cares if the place is salvaged? After all, in a big city, when a hospital closes, other hospitals just pick up the slack.

At Baptist, we decided to try to create a unique and special culture of caring. This, we hoped, would be a place where people truly tried to live out the mission statement. Subsequently, we named it The New Healing Hospital. In January, 2001, we formally introduced the concept to the staff at Baptist. They already understood we were just putting a new name on something we had been working to develop for years — a job that continues to this day.

In the midst of recovering from the massive "tornado-like" damage of a 73-million-dollar loss, we decided not to do some of the most obvious things. We followed the guidance of the "Rings of Care" and decided to hire more nurses instead of cutting hundreds of frontline caregivers. We also asked ourselves several hard questions about why we were needed in the Nashville community and what, if anything, was unique about our services. No one could recite the current mission statement. Like many, it was too long and cumbersome. We dusted off the mission statement (literally as well as figuratively) and launched a one-year inquiry into what our mission statement should be.

Work like this never succeeds unless you have an outstanding team of leaders. Under the direction of our exquisite Medical Staff President at the time, Keith Hagan, M.D., and our gifted new Senior Vice President, Tracy Wimberly, R.N., who came with me from Ohio, we began this lengthy inquiry. Paul Moore, the long-time and capable Chief Operating Officer at Baptist, played a key role, as did Debby Koch, our talented and dedicated communications Vice President. Susan Crutchfield helped us with her extensive experience with the services side of the organization. Later, two other gifted leaders, Jeff Kaplan and Stephanie Zembar, joined us, and subsequent to all of this, we got the great services of Jim O'Keefe to serve as Chief Financial Officer and Deke Ellwanger to head up managed care. Each provided invaluable help as we moved to rid ourselves of trouble, negotiate with other hospitals, and focus on moving the organization forward to live out its mission.

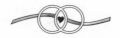

Ultimately, our success at Baptist from 1998 to 2002 did not come merely from making budget cuts. It was the concept and practice of the Healing Hospital that turned the place around. That is because the application of loving leadership that is integral to the Healing Hospital released the great strengths of leaders and caregivers who were already present in the organization. Like the gift of the Magi that is part of the Christian tradition, Healing Hospital leadership discovers and releases the gifts that are already present in any organization.

Across the years we learned that the culture of a Healing Hospital pays deep respect to processes and relationships. In developing our mission statement, the final words we arrived at may not be as important as 1) the respectful way in which we involved the staff, and 2) the fact that we kept the final statement short and memorable.

Below is the mission statement we came up with together. Due to a respectful response from the new owners of Baptist and its fine mission officer, Julie O'Connor, this mission statement remains a part of Baptist to this day. Here are its fourteen words:

We are a caring community, devoted to healing
with love in the Christian tradition.[52]

The challenge of the Healing Hospital is that some people will persistently doubt that this model can succeed. They will have many opportunities to undermine this work because this model takes a while to "kick in." They will continue to try to derail the loving, healing agenda in favor of short-term financial fixes. But both the Baptist story and the story of Riverside Methodist Hospital and the OhioHealth system in Columbus prove that the healing care agenda can bring outstanding financial success and other great outcomes across the organization.

THE DOCK, THE BOAT, AND IN BETWEEN

The foundation needs to be laid for a whole new pattern of leadership training to gain the support of middle management, to give them the tools to do the job, and to find out who's not willing to get on board with the change. For this change at Baptist, I continually used the example of a person going from a dock onto a rowboat.

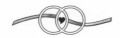

There are three choices: you can stay on the dock, you can get in the boat, or you can be in that awkward spot in between with one foot on the dock and the other on the boat. It's possible to be in that third spot briefly — but not for long. At some point everyone has either got to get into the boat or stay on the dock, because the boat is leaving.

> *What would your hospital be like if every caregiver behaved as a kind and loving person?*

Interestingly, one hundred percent of the audiences I question say they believe in loving care. Rarely does anyone claim they practice this belief one hundred percent of the time. We are simply asking people to live out what they already believe, and for organizations to do the same. What's radical about all this is the idea that every caregiver can be loving in his or her work. What would that look like? What would your hospital be like if every caregiver behaved as a kind and loving person?

Most American hospitals have not yet been successful in creating environments of loving care. The work of the Healing Hospital strives to address this problem by offering a new and aggressive model on which to bring about revelatory change.

This model will work if leadership makes a deep commitment to it over the years, not just for a few weeks and months. Pervasive loving cultures cannot be established in a short time. The first goal of the Healing Hospital is to establish healing environments for the legions of our fellow caregivers who are walking the hallways of our hospitals often feeling distrustful of leadership and burned out at their jobs.

It is leadership's job to lift up a new vision — to literally love the caregivers so they may be free to give love to patients. Meaning is healing. Leaders who offer exciting visions to their organizations and follow them up with real action can heal burnout by energizing their staff.

LIFE MAGIC!

I believe that our life begins when we begin the work we were meant to do. This is work we truly love — not only because it is joyful, but also because it is the way we can best serve others. When caregivers are caring for patients (and each other) with love, the result is to put in place forces that will reveal magic that is already there. Magic rises up from a commitment to God's

> *Meaning is healing.*

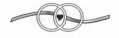

work and a willingness to be present to the miracles that are already before us each day. With a passionate life commitment and an open heart, magic will begin to appear. Our responsibility is to go deeper. This commitment is captured exquisitely in the last stanza of my favorite Robert Frost poem, "Two Tramps in Mud Time," which I print again here:

> *My object in living is to unite*
> *My avocation and my vocation*
> *As my two eyes make one in sight*
> *Only where love and need are one,*
> *And the work is play for mortal stakes,*
> *Is the deed ever really done*
> *For heaven and the future's sakes.*

Magic appears when we learn to become present to the world — to learn to see and hear with sacred eyes and ears the miracles that have already been placed here by God. Since God is present, then magic is as well. When we commit to make love and need one and work becomes "play for mortal stakes," we are putting in place the conditions for magic to appear to us, not only in stories but real life where we begin to learn, as Professor Patout Burns said once to me, that "the myths are true."

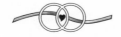

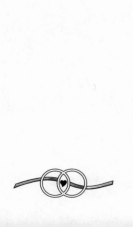

Chapter 3

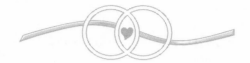

CULTIVATING A CULTURE
OF SACRED WORK

CULTURE SHIFT AND WAVE THEORY

Once about a quarter of the partners in a new hospital culture are deeply committed to loving care, it will be seen that the rest of the organization has quietly started migrating the same way. The wave has begun to move, in an all-important culture shift. This movement may seem as slow and subtle as a glacier, but it will be perceptible on close examination. As a leader, you need to announce this change and encourage it. That will speed the movement.

Accept the fact that there will always be a hard core at the cynical end of the spectrum. But the majority will act the same way you and I acted on our first day of school. In kindergarten, when you and I started school, one of the first things we did was to look around at the other kids and at the teachers to see how things were done. If people were friendly, we acted friendly. If people seemed mean, we tried to act tough. Probably three-quarters of employees are the same way. When the culture wave starts to surge in a particular direction, most will adapt to the new temperature of the water.

The power of this phenomenon is crucial to understanding both organizational and team culture. Positive teams naturally influence new members toward positive behavior. Negative teams do the same, but toward negative behavior. This is the reason a positive team leader is so critical. He or she sets the tone and can, over time, create an environment that will emphasize the right values.

It is important to be both patient and persistent in this process. It may often feel as slow as turning around an aircraft carrier — but when the ship is turned, it becomes a great vessel headed in the right direction.

Wave Theory® in Visionary Change

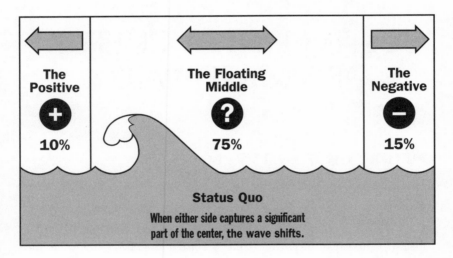

Momentum shifts in a predictable manner I call "Wave Theory." Wave theory is encouraging in that *it demonstrates that moving a culture is easier than many believe.* It is discouraging in that the culture can swing *back* in the opposite direction absent supportive leadership. Over the past three decades I have seen both ends of the phenomenon in organizations I have led. Some further words of warning in this regard may be helpful, with a couple of stories.

RIVERSIDE METHODIST HOSPITAL

In 1983, I took over as President and CEO of the largest (1000 beds) hospital in Ohio, Riverside Methodist in Columbus. The hospital had been competently run in a traditional manner. The bottom line was small but stable. In spite of its size, the hospital had a flat profile outside of Columbus. Essentially, it was seen as a good but not great community hospital.

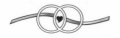

How do you wake up a hospital that is doing okay, but not great? A suggestion for significant change will always be met by skeptics who say something like, "Hey, things are going fine, why change?" and that tiresome old saw, "If it ain't broke, don't fix it."

The best answer I have heard for cynics like this is something I will paraphrase from Tom Peters. Someone apparently asked him in a meeting why he was pushing so hard and finally said to Peters, "Why are you pushing us so hard, we're no worse than anyone else." To which Peters responded, "Oh, now there's a great slogan for a company — buy our products, we're no worse than anyone else."

This is exactly what I was trying to say to cynics at Riverside Methodist in the early 1980s. We posed a series of questions: Do we want to send our mothers to a hospital that is just okay? Do we want to work for one of America's most okay hospitals?

Where is the passion for excellence in a situation like this? Passion always lives a long way away from mediocrity. To me, accepting a lukewarm status quo is equivalent to admitting mediocrity. It is unethical to settle for average when you could be great.

Riverside Methodist clearly had the potential to be way above "just okay." Our team there launched a pattern of new initiatives to strengthen the culture clinically, organizationally, economically, and most of all, spiritually. We developed a new vision of excellence and a cardinal value that we would honor the dignity and worth of each person.

RIVERSIDE MAGIC

Magical outcomes arise from the *realization* of dreams, not their conceptualization. It is important to understand that the magic is always there, waiting for leaders to discover it and reveal it. Here's the happy bottom line: The Riverside Methodist story is remarkably similar to the Baptist Hospital System story. Both successes represent the enormous power of magic when the forces of the Healing Hospital concept are put into place.

In 1983, Riverside was a single hospital with a bottom line of about 2 million dollars. Twelve years later, Riverside Methodist had become the flagship for the eight-hospital OhioHealth System. The system bottom line (FY '95) was over 56 million dollars![53]

Clinically, across twelve years of Healing Hospital–style leadership, Riverside made dramatic improvements in our Centers of Excellence in heart, cancer, and woman's health. The heart program, under Jeff Kaplan's

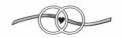

leadership, became one of the top in the country. The cancer program developed as a Regional Center of Excellence, and the women's health program, under Tracy Wimberly, expanded to the point where the Riverside system was clearly the leader in the state with over nine thousand births per year.

To achieve magical results like this, a great team is always essential. With the leadership of Tracy Wimberly, Riverside developed one of the top ten hospice programs in the country. In Mark Evans, we had at OhioHealth the best Human Resources leader. He developed a spectacular employee relations program that placed Riverside among the most employee-friendly hospitals in the country. We were also fortunate to have Jeff Kaplan as a world-class fundraiser. With his leadership, the foundation grew from about 2 million dollars to over 50 million, and also resulted in the development of the nationally renowned McConnell Health Care Center. We had excellence as well in the leadership of Nick Baird, M.D., as our Medical Director.

The rest of the all-star team included Bill Wilkins and Frank Pandora, who guided our efforts at merging seven more hospitals into our system. We never actually had to "pay" for one of them, although we assumed debt responsibilities in some cases. Either we convinced them they would be more successful if they joined our system, or they decided on their own that the OhioHealth bandwagon was the one to join. We had exceptional leadership in patient care services from Marian Hamm, M.S.N., who developed one of the finest nursing programs in the country. Steve Garlock oversaw a widely successful communications campaign. Bill and Dave Blom led the remarkable turnaround of Grant Hospital after it joined our system. In addition, we had a highly competent leader at Riverside in Nancy Schlichting. Nancy was first Chief Operating Officer with me and was subsequently President at Riverside. She did an especially effective job of working with the medical staff.

There is typically a close relationship between a magical leadership team and employee satisfaction and patient satisfaction. Satisfied employees do not, as some believe, become lazy. Instead, they raise their commitment to making patients happy as well. Of course the reverse is also true. In 1983, patient and employee satisfaction had been at satisfactory but not exceptional levels.

By 1995, patient satisfaction had soared and employee satisfaction was so high that Riverside was selected as a top-three hospital (along with Boston's Beth Israel and the famed Mayo Clinic) in Ron Zemke's Service

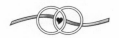

America. Riverside was also described as a top-ten hospital when it was featured on the ABC special "Revolution at Work" with Forrest Sawyer. And it was highlighted as one of the best places to work in America in *Working Mother Magazine*. Mark Evans advised me in late 1994 that we had 30,000 applications over the past year for only 800 jobs!

When partners see great results like this, they start to want to live up to them. These outcomes really helped move the culture wave in the right direction for Riverside in Columbus. It's like when I was a little kid and I hit my sister. My mother said to me, "I'm surprised at you. You are a nice boy, you don't hit your sister." I remember thinking to myself, "Well, maybe she's right. If I am a nice boy I guess I wouldn't hit my sister." I wanted to live up to the label my mother gave me, so I stopped hitting my sister. Employee partners want to live up to the reputation of the hospital of which they are a part.

> *When partners see great results ... they start wanting to live up to them*

We know that we often respond to the labels others give us. If we think we're no good at math, we may not even try very hard to be good. If we think we're part of an uncaring and failed organization, we may stop caring ourselves. And we may start to give up in our work. This, of course, is a damaging syndrome. Accordingly, a strong reputation should favorably affect the performance and productivity of most caregivers.

WHAT COULD GO WRONG?
A REVERSE CULTURE SHIFT

In the face of all this success, what could go wrong? I offer the following example as an illustration of how negative forces can damage a Healing Hospital initiative, even when it has been firmly put in place for several years. For sadly, in early 1995, after *twelve consecutive years of steadily rising success*, some of our board members got anxious when a consultant warned about a managed care invasion from California. Pressure on me to radically cut costs began to build, even though the hospital had just recorded a booming profit of 56 million dollars on $800 million in revenues. At one point, the consultant offered a formula: Cut 1000 employees and $100 million dollars in 18 months.[54]

For a non-profit organization with a fat bottom line, this seemed to me ridiculous. I warned that if this kind of action were taken, morale would plummet and the organization might tail downward. There were other

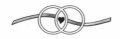

issues brewing at the time as well, but pretty soon the notion spread that, after twelve years, maybe I had overstayed my welcome. Maybe I wasn't "mean enough" to make the radical cuts some thought were necessary. Maybe it was time for a new leader.

Ultimately, under great pressure, I agreed. When you discover that some board members who have followed you for twelve years suddenly seem to have gone deaf to your leadership and you can't find a new way to connect with them, it's time to leave. An amicable separation was worked out and our successful experience at Riverside/OhioHealth came to a heartbreaking end.

It's remarkable how non-profit boards of trustees can sometimes be like the owners of a baseball team. The team wins the World Series and then the owner starts selling off players and tinkering with the team as if it were an auto engine needing an adjustment. Once I left, the rest of our spectacular team started to come apart. Person after person eventually departed and the magic began to vanish.

My personal view was that this happened because I was unwilling to make the drastic cuts in the way they were offered. Perhaps they were right — I am not mean enough, or foolish enough, to lay people off when the hospital is generating a huge bottom line. I believed that a more gradual restructuring would have preserved the culture of committed employees and that drastic cuts would kill morale, create confusion, and lead to losses.

Unfortunately, I turned out to be right about this. For the first year after I left, a positive financial picture was sustained. I am advised that soon, however, the organization fell into the red. To the deep dismay of many, this red ink triggered a round of severe employee layoffs. This included what I consider to be a particularly disastrous decision when, in the later part of 1997, hundreds of staff were let go in the kind of bloodbath that all employees fear. The damage caused by a layoff like this is seen by the horror stories that quickly emerged. These were stories of loyal long-term employees being fired and taken to their cars by security officers.

It is rare for staff to be strong enough to speak out to top-level leaders in the midst of savage actions like this. Most people are either intimidated or think their actions won't matter. One senior nurse, Rita Smith, R.N., to her enduring credit, had the courage to approach a senior board member to tell him, to his surprise, that she would never forgive him for supporting such a terrible action. Rita is a person who respects the tradition and history of Riverside. She knows injustice when she sees it. She is one of those invaluable team members who has the integrity to speak up for the

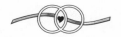

best values of an organization she loves and to which she has dedicated her worklife.

Needless to say, the layoff did *not* bring a meaningful turnaround. Instead, things got worse. As any good CEO might have predicted, morale went south and the organization entered a downward spiral. I am told that there were four more years of consecutive losses until new leadership was appointed in 2001.

For an organization that had been doing so well, how could this have happened? Why wouldn't OhioHealth have continued with the team that had led so successfully for twelve straight years? It's difficult for me to say — or perhaps to even be objective about it. But clearly, Riverside and OhioHealth had developed a Healing Hospital culture before we had a name for it. Although we had this culture in the flagship hospital of the system, we had not fully extended it to the board itself. And we had not planned for succession.

Again, I cite this example as a warning that the garden that is the Healing Hospital needs constant tending. There will always be those who wish to destroy it or who think another gardener can do better. Volunteer boards can be very difficult to manage over long periods, and I was probably overconfident about the degree to which they would understand the day-to-day culture of the organization and the enormous importance of trying to protect and preserve this culture. One particularly difficult board member did not, in my view, understand what a great success we had until after he had helped engineer my departure. As the organization went into a negative spiral, he said to me a couple of years later that the time of my leadership had been the "glory days" — a time of Camelot-type success. In this same conversation, he feigned innocence over any role he might have played in causing the negative change. Meanwhile, the CEO that presided over this decline had been an outstanding Chief Financial Officer. Unfortunately, success as a finance officer does not automatically translate to success as a CEO.

> *Negative leadership generates negative results.*

Some people think fear-based leadership scares people into peak performance. My theory is simply that, with time, negative leadership generates negative results. It appears that the approach of the new leader resulted in a deterioration of the loving culture of the organization.

Numerous people complained that the replacement leadership had

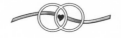

never effectively offered a hopeful vision. One senior leader said to me, "After you, we got a person who was a good finance guy, but there was no compelling vision."

The additional point of all this is to demonstrate both the positive and negative possibilities revealed by the Wave Theory in cultural change. When the positive wave rises, it can lift and move the entire organization to the shores of success. When the momentum turns negative, however, the wave shifts and the results can be disastrous. Boards of trust have a high responsibility to protect against shifts to the negative and to ensure the presence of positive leadership that can reverse these shifts as quickly as possible.

> *Boards of trust have a high responsibility to protect against shifts to the negative and to ensure the presence of positive leadership that can reverse these shifts as quickly as possible.*

One of the great challenges of Radical Loving Care in a Healing Hospital is that it invites people to trust each other and their leaders. As long as this trust is honored, great strides can be made because partners will bring forward their very best efforts and their very best ideas. When this trust is dishonored through savage and unnecessary layoffs done with police-style tactics, partners become mere employees again. Many will begin to offer minimum effort and save their ideas for other settings.

Yet another leadership team has now taken over at OhioHealth, and the reports I have are that this team is doing a better job of re-centering the organization on the right values. Among other things, the current CEO has been complimented for listening to his staff and employees. Perhaps he will yet be the kind of servant leader that can offer the kind of compelling vision that will return that organization to the ranks of a true Healing Hospital where loving care is the hallmark. Meanwhile, with the leadership change, the organization has apparently returned to profitability as of fiscal year 2003.[55] The embers of the Healing Hospital culture of loving care remain at Riverside Methodist and can be re-ignited. The biggest risk for OhioHealth, as for any successful organization, is that they will be lulled by what author Jim Collins calls in his book *Good to Great* the obstacle of being good rather than great. Good organizations, Collins claims, often become complacent. This complacency causes them to falter. Along the pathway to greatness, they stop for a time in the comfort zone of being good and decide the rest of the way requires too much effort. This is the great obstacle blocking Healing Hospital implementation in so many

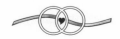

places. It's just too hard for most organizations to sustain the high effort required to truly reach the summit of loving service.

Mr. Collins also emphasizes another point with which I agree. The positive culture of an organization must never be too dependent on a single leader. This was a mistake I apparently made at Riverside and OhioHealth that I regret. If I had done a better job of implanting the culture of loving care with the board, perhaps they might have made wiser choices after I left. Perhaps this illustration will serve as a caution against tying a Healing Hospital culture too tightly to one person.

PEER POWER: THE MILGRAM EXPERIMENT, THE STANFORD PRISON EXPERIMENT, AND GROUPTHINK IN WAVE THEORY

In the early 1960s, psychologist Stanley Milgram developed and oversaw a series of experiments that are now famous.[56] A series of subjects were told they were participating in a study to determine how people learn. They were seated at a mock "shock generator" in front of a series of switches that supposedly applied increasing amounts of electric shocks. Each subject was instructed to administer shocks to an unseen person in the next room whenever the person made a mistake in reciting a certain memory sequence. As the mistakes increased, the subject was ordered by a lab-coated instructor to administer higher and higher levels of shocks — from slight (15 volts) up to dangerous (450 volts). As the shocks increased, the unseen victim would scream out louder and louder in apparent pain.

Remarkably, two-thirds of the subjects administered the highest level of shocks when ordered to do so! This led Milgram to conclude that when people are ordered to do something by an authority figure, most of them will obey *even though it directly violates their personal values.*

Though the experiment was designed in part to explain the reaction of Germans to Nazi rule, it has an interesting application in Wave Theory and our study of Healing Hospitals. Like the Milgram Experiment, Wave Theory suggests the effect of one group of humans on another. In Wave Theory, employees are not only influenced by instructions from their bosses, but by the behavior of their peers. Loving environments promote loving behavior. Fear-driven environments promote defensive and paranoid behaviors.

A particularly dramatic example of the impact of fear-driven behaviors is demonstrated in the Stanford Prison Experiment,[56] in which volunteers

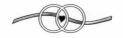

were placed in simulated roles as prisoners and guards. The experiment was so powerful that it had to be interrupted on the sixth day because volunteer guards had gotten carried away with the power of their roles and volunteer prisoners had become effectively intimidated.

Groupthink, a concept developed by Irving Janis, advances the notion that individuals in certain decision groups will start to default to the opinion of the group in order to be amicable.[58] Pressures in this kind of environment can be so strong that individuals may be unwilling to share opinions that differ from the majority for fear of being rejected.

Each of these studies demonstrates the enormous impact of peer pressure. Peer behaviors in all cultures are enormously powerful in driving individual behaviors. This is certainly true in the hierarchical environment of hospitals. Patients suffer in fear-driven employee cultures because employees are less likely to act lovingly if they are not being loved themselves. Conversely, in environments where employee partners are treated with love and respect, patients are much more likely to receive loving care.

ANOTHER CULTURAL KEY IN A HEALING HOSPITAL: THE PROCESSES OF DIALOGUE, INQUIRY, AND PILOTING

At the outset of this work, the processes of dialogue, inquiry, and piloting were emphasized as a prerequisite. That is because these processes are by far the most effective way to learn. We remember only a little bit of what we hear and not much of what we read. We learn things better when we can discover them through a process of inquiry. If I tell you how to give loving care, how will you feel? Probably somewhat resentful. If I ask you how you give loving care, then you will explain the answer to me. In so doing, you will become a teacher and you will be more likely to want to practice what you are teaching. After all, you are now a professor on loving care in your particular area.

Start thinking about the kinds of questions that would provoke the change you seek in your world. Questions directed at asking others how they accomplish certain kinds of success are questions that inherently honor the other person. These questions can also be reframed to take performance up another step. I will pose a question like this to you: If you had to improve the level of loving care on your team or in your area, how would you do it?

I strongly recommend the use of piloting as a way to test new ideas in

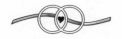

a large organization. Remember that piloting can be limited in time as well as size of area where the idea is piloted. If the ER wants to test putting a direct caregiver at the front entrance instead of an admitting clerk, try it for a while on the day shift to see how it goes. There will usually be resistance to a new system. Beware of giving up too quickly. Give the pilot a chance to work. Make notes. Make adjustments. Most of all, stay committed to the idea that things can be improved and that improvement will happen with your teams.

RIPPLE POWER

God will not shield us from the journey, but God will support us through the journey.

— Michelle Jackson

A law of physics is that for each action, there is an equal and opposite reaction. In human behavior, for each action there is always an effect, like the ripple that goes out when a pebble is tossed into a lake. The Ripple Effect is one of the most beautiful elements of God's magic. The concept is suggested by comments from the late Senator Robert Kennedy about the way in which our actions send out ripples into the world. It is also a concept I have seen successfully used in a beautiful community service organization, City Year, founded in Boston by Alan Khazei and Michael Brown.

Dr. James Sullivan, co-founder of Baptist Hospital in 1948, said to me once that "our best deeds, we do unknowingly." This means that we may do a kind act that will change the lives of people we never see. The importance of all this is for us to accept that, even though we may not see the outcome, our actions, good or bad, have effects. The hit-and-run driver may never know the way in which he or she has ruined the life of a victim. The anonymous Good Samaritan may also never know how much his or her kindness has transformed the life of another.

It's A Wonderful Life is one of the most popular movies of all time. Perhaps it is because we are all enchanted by the notion that our life has meaning and that meaning may be found in the way we affect the lives of others. Knowing about the Ripple Effect can help leaders and partners understand how powerful their positive actions can be.

For years I have been sending flowers anonymously to elderly patients

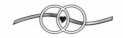

who are identified by staff members as patients who may be needful. The card usually says simply, "From someone who cares about you." I never know what effect this has on a particular patient, but it is likely that this small act creates a Ripple Effect that brings waves of joy to many lonely people.

MARTHA'S RIPPLES!

Consider my younger sister, Martha. Martha was born with something called achondroplasia, a type of dwarfism. But as my father often said about her, her spirit is ten feet tall. Each day at the information desk at The Toledo Hospital, she commits acts of kindness that ripple through the lives of others. For example, each morning for many years, Martha has said "hello" to everyone she passes — whether they respond or not. One Christmas she was surprised to receive a note and a gift from a shy employee who had never once returned Martha's hundreds of cheerful morning greetings. The note said, "Thank you, Martha, you will never know how much your morning greetings have meant to me. Sorry I've always been too shy to respond."

This is one example of thanks this Good Samaritan received for her kindness. But for every single thank you, there are hundreds of other kindnesses that have rippled out from her Servant's Heart that have had wonderful effects of which she will never know. Unconditional love always offers kindness with no expectation of repayment.

At a Healing Hospital, we constantly preach the importance of saying hello to strangers and of helping people who look lost to find their way. We also talk about "little" things like how cleanliness is next to godliness, and that it's important to pick up paper off the floor because "we're all caregivers" and "we're all housekeepers."

These things seem small and their ripples will always be hard to measure. Still, the ripples from our kind acts can have remote and beautiful consequences. We need to do these things because they are right, not because we expect a reward. When partners practice Ripple Power, morale goes up — and so does patient and family satisfaction. The wave of the hospital's culture begins to move toward the shoreline of the positive.

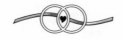

Summary of the Elements of Ripple Power

- The Servant's Heart offers love unconditionally. It sends forth a "ripple" into the universe.

- Our kind and loving acts have remote and extensive consequences we may never see and cannot imagine.

- Knowing about the "ripple effect" encourages the heart of a servant and moves the culture wave toward positive waters.

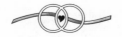

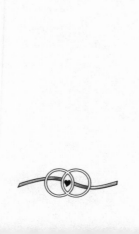

Chapter 4

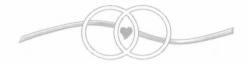

THE SACRED ENCOUNTER
IN PRACTICE

*You have to be a blessing to give a blessing. So I ask God to bless me
each morning so that I may be a blessing to my patients.*
— Deadre Hall, R.N., Critical Care Nurse

Deadre Hall has been asking God to bless her every morning for
twenty-five years before she heads off to work caring for the critically ill at Baptist Hospital. She does this because she knows her
patients need healing from her. They need her clinical skills, and they need
for her to give her gifts in a loving way. "I don't need to bring my problems
into the patient's room. That patient has his own problems. I need to open
up my heart to that patient's needs," she says. She also understands how
hard the work is — both emotionally and physically.

Fortunately, the practice of Sacred Encounters does not require white-
hot intensity across the day. A helpful way to think about love's expression
in these encounters is, perhaps, to think of them in stages or levels.
Consider the intent that underlies each of our actions. Do we enter each
day with love, or is our intent to squeeze from each day the maximum gain
for ourselves?

It continues to be important that we distinguish the Sacred Encounter
from the transaction meetings that infect and weaken so much of our lives.

Again, transactional encounters are those we do to fulfill everyday needs. Ordinary daily encounters may fall into some portion of the simple grid on the left; the examples are there simply as illustrations. The grid on the right illustrates how our encounters may be graphed in a hospital context.

The Encounter Window

	Random	Planned
Brief	Paying Cashier	Buying Gas
Prolonged	Irish Pub	Marriage

	Random	Planned
Brief	Cafeteria Cashier	Hospital
Prolonged	Severe Accident	Rehab. Therapy

Our daily interpersonal interactions can be meaningful or not, and they can be intimate or not, depending on the critical components of love and need and the intentions of those in the encounter. The brevity and randomness of an encounter do not necessarily control its meaning or intimacy. A brief random encounter with a cashier who happens to be Lois Powers may be meaningful if the cashier happens to reach out in a kind way to us at a time we are feeling particularly vulnerable. A marriage, on the other hand, may be both planned and prolonged, but could conceivably hold little meaning. If both partners simply go through the motions as if it were a series of transactions and neither really commits the heart to the marriage, than how meaningful and intimate is it, even if it is lengthy?

In a patient care context, it is the joining of love with need that can infuse each encounter with meaning, *even if the encounter is both brief and random.* The story of Lois Powers, the loving cashier at Baptist, is a strong illustration of this. Almost every one of Lois's encounters as a cashier was brief. This is true almost by definition, since Lois would not be demonstrating loving service to delay her line of customers with a prolonged discussion with one client. As we all know, most cashiers don't try to engage us very much. There's no time. Except that Lois always tried to bring light into the lives of each person with a little joke or a light touch on the arm and a smile. Her intent was to be "a caregiver, not a cashier." Who can calculate the impact of Lois's kindness on her endless string of customers?

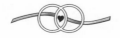

Most other cashiers are engaged in mere transactions. Because of both her intent and her actions, Lois engaged in the practice of Sacred Encounters with each customer. So long as love informs our actions, each of our daily meetings can be transformed from a transaction into a Sacred Encounter of some importance on the continuum illustrated below.

The chance for deeper encounters is somewhat more likely in the prolonged and planned relationship between a nurse and a terminally ill cancer patient. Here the concept of presence is particularly acute. Cancer patients may be highly attuned to the demeanor of the nurse as soon as she or he enters the room. Is this more bad news? Are you going to give me another painful treatment? Or are you here to comfort me?

The degree to which love can transform each encounter may be understood on a chart that indicates a progression in intimacy and meaning.

Highest Level of Sacred Encounter

Where Deep Need Meets Deep Love

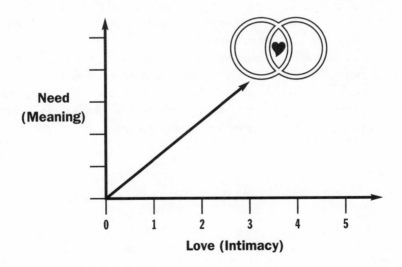

The actual need for love and the way in which it is most effectively given can never be precisely placed on any kind of graph. The goal of this chart, however, is to suggest that as the need of a patient increases, there should be a parallel increase in the love that will meet the need. The greater

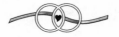

the need for loving care, the greater the demand on the caregiver to provide the loving care. When love actually does keep rising to meet increasing need, then the intensity of the encounter is likely to rise as well.

This is the reason we so often reference examples like the housekeeper and the old man or the nurse and the dying baby in the stories told earlier. The baby cannot express its need to be held and comforted in its dying moments, yet we can imagine that the need is great and the nurse is successfully rising to meet it. A nurse who feels that part of the job is to comfort the dying as well as to support the living has added a whole new dimension of meaning to her or his work.

Parallel, but more obvious examples of the effort of love to meet need occurs in the film *Sacred Work*,[59] which tells the stories of some Sacred Encounters at Baptist Hospital. In one sequence, a patient is crying out with unimaginable pain. His cry seems to signal not only physical pain but fear, loneliness, and sadness all in one. The nurses are barred from giving further relief medication because of the delicate nature of the patient's condition. Instead, they simply stand by him and stroke his arm and hold his hand and struggle to soothe him with the soft instruments of their voices. They seem like two mothers trying to calm a crying baby — except that this is a full-grown man in exquisite pain. Still, one of them even refers to him as "baby," reinforcing how clearly she understands this patient's deep need for the loving comfort of a mother.

In many hospitals, patients with intractable pain like this are literally just left to suffer. Nurses sometimes write these patients off as delirious and beyond soothing. This is deeply disturbing because it is so unnecessary. No suffering patient should be left alone, and in a Healing Hospital, no patient is left beyond the efforts of caregivers to offer comfort.

Chapter 5

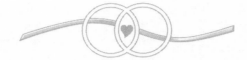

REQUIRED LEADERSHIP STYLE

Neither a lofty degree of intelligence nor imagination nor both together go to the making of genius. Love, love, love, that is the soul of genius.

— Wolfgang Amadeus Mozart

WHERE IS LOVE ON THE LEADERSHIP AGENDA?

It's easy to see the effects of raw power when it's misused, as when terrified people are being shoved around by an overbearing leader. It's somewhat harder to see the effects of loving leadership. But as Mozart said, and as he proved with his astonishing array of brilliant music, love is the soul of genius. Employee partners who are loved by leaders clearly care more about their work. The tyrant trusts no one and therefore must use force to get results. The loving leader offers a strong vision and trusts people to do their best to meet that vision. He or she knows how to wait patiently for the good results that generally come from loving leadership.

Tyranny fails to appreciate other people as human. This can manifest itself in a leader who thinks of employees as units of expense. Autocrats tend to see every person as replaceable, when in fact the job is what is replaceable, not the person. No person, good or bad, can ever be replaced,

139

even though their position can be filled with someone else.

How do we know that love has departed from the center of hospital care? Look at the agenda of almost any leaders meeting, doctors meeting, or board meeting. The best most groups do with love on the agenda is to open with a devotional message. Some may also have a little time devoted to "mission." But following the devotional, the leader of the meeting will typically say something like, "Thank you for the devotional, now let's get to our business . . . " It's almost as if the leader had said, "Now that we've got that soft stuff out of the way, let's move on to the stuff that *really* counts!"

> *The purpose of the Healing Hospital movement is to change the agenda of American healthcare...*

The signal here is obvious: love doesn't seem to merit much attention from leaders, doctors, or board members. Lest we all become defensive about this, I don't think this happens because these groups don't care about love. What is more likely, *they don't know exactly what to say*. The purpose of the Healing Hospital movement is to change the agenda of American healthcare so that all decisions are love-based and mission weaves its way throughout the agenda.

WHAT'S HAPPENING ON THE FRONT LINES?

Meanwhile, what's happening out on the front lines? Imagine our familiar example of the ER admitting clerk. You enter the Emergency department of a major hospital with a pain in your side and you struggle up to the admitting desk. What will the admitting clerk say? You already know. "Name? Address? Insurance card?" Leadership, through its insensitivity and wrong focus, has signaled to her and to admitting clerks all over America that *their role is only to collect information*. What if she could take a few seconds more to express some concern and to greet you as a human being? Some clerks do this, of course, but it is clearly not seen as a part of their job. Frontline staff are not being supported in their desire to give care that is loving as well as efficient.

The purpose of the Healing Hospital movement is to change the agenda of American healthcare so that love returns to its rightful place at the center. This movement seeks to open a new pathway that will illuminate the role love must play in all of healthcare — particularly in hospitals, at the bedside of the acutely ill patient.

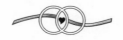

There are dramatic arrays of ongoing initiatives in most major hospitals that will take colossal forward steps when leaders embrace and support the Healing Hospital culture. Consider the vast agenda of patient safety issues that are so critical to the ongoing health of patients. What is most likely to motivate reduced medication errors? Will it be a supervisor who threatens and intimidates his or her staff, or will it be a motivated group of employee partners who decide giving the right medication is the best way to give loving care?

Most patient safety issues do not depend on acquiring new technology as much as they depend on the motivation of the people using the technology. Operator error is a far bigger concern than equipment malfunction. If employee motivation is the key to solving even half the issues, then the obvious solution for leaders is to consider how best to motivate employees. This is the core of the appeal of the Healing Hospital to leaders. Healing Hospitals are safer because the partners in these hospitals care so deeply about their patients that they will use their best efforts to ensure premier care. And this is why the Healing Hospital is vital to the future of American healthcare. Motivation matters. Leaders need to commit themselves to the selection, training, and support of motivated work forces who are affirmed in every way possible by top leadership. This doesn't mean speeches, it means consistent presence on the front lines, competitive wages and benefits, and a positive working environment.

This is the kind of leadership displayed by enlightened people like Jim Nathan, President and CEO of Lee Memorial in Fort Myers, Florida. Jim served an extensive and highly successful term as head of this hospital system, took an extended break to enhance his skills, then returned to Lee Memorial recently to lead them back to top performance again. His deep and sincere commitment to peak performance for every aspect of his organization has distinguished his hospital and has made it a more healing place. Jim knows how to lead through both example and presence, and this is why he is successful.

The same is true of Elaine Ullian, President and CEO of Boston Medical Center. Elaine has led with energy and vigor and the utmost integrity in the face of the enormous challenges of running a big-city academic medical center. Her organization delivers exceptional care to an extraordinarily diverse group of patients, and Elaine provides world-class leadership to her organization as it competes in the shadow of the several Harvard teaching hospitals. She succeeds not by focusing on the competition but by giving her heart and soul to the employees she leads and the

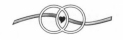

doctors she works with.

I must highlight, again, the exceptional leadership of Hank Walker, former President and CEO of Providence Health System based in Seattle, and Dennis Vonderfecht, President and CEO of Mountain States Health System in Johnson City, Tennessee. Hank is a person of deep spirituality. His rich and beautiful commitment to healing healthcare continues to be reflected in the enlightened pathway of his system in establishing healing work. Dennis has launched a Healing Hospital initiative across his eight-hospital system and has appointed two people to serve as Healing Hospital officers for his system. It is only through steps like the ones Dennis is taking that a Healing Hospital can truly take hold, and he is to be especially commended for his pioneering work. Indeed, on a two-day visit through several of the hospitals in the Mountain States System, I was startled at how effective his leadership has already been. Staff in the Mountain States hospitals demonstrate an extraordinarily high level of caring and innovation and both staff morale and patient satisfaction are high.

Examples of leaders like these, along with Mike Stephens at Hoag Memorial Hospital in Newport Beach; Gary Mecklenburg at Northwestern University Hospital, Chicago; Nancy Schlichting at Henry Ford Health System in Detroit; Tom Priselac at Cedars Sinai in Los Angeles; Martha Marsh at Stanford University Hospital; Joe Zaccagnino at Yale-New Haven Hospital; Gary Strack at Boca Raton Community Hospital; and Mike Means at Health First in Melbourne, Florida, give hope to all of us that American healthcare can change for the better.

One of the things every great leader is always watching for is the employee partner who has a Servant's Heart. Perhaps we all wonder how this kind of person is created. When I would look into the warm and compassionate eyes of Baptist Hospital Chaplain Michelle Jackson, I used to wonder from where the love in those eyes came. I suppose the answer would be from her heart. But upon looking into her heart, my guess is that we would have been directed back to her eyes. The eyes reflect the heart and a caring heart is always reflected through the eyes and the hands. A servant knows how to listen through the eyes and a servant knows not only how to touch a patient but, of equal importance, *whether* to touch that patient.

In most people, the Servant's Heart is present but is waiting for the encouragement of leaders to fully express itself. Leaders with a Servant's Heart are always able to identify others who have the same capability. For example, the Servant's Heart of a great nurse leader like Nancy Moore at

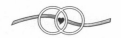

Saint Charles Hospital in Bend, Oregon, is the reason that the patient care staff there contains so many wonderful servants. The level of Servanthood in a hospital or charity is typically a reflection of the degree to which the top leadership are true servants. And most leaders do have a Servant's Heart themselves. With some, that heart is buried so deep down it's hard to tell that its there. With others, as mentioned above, that caring heart is very evident.

MAGI TRAINING AND HIGH PURPOSE LEADERSHIP

We live the whole of our lives provisionally. We think that for the time being things are bad, that for the time being we must make the best of them and adapt or humiliate ourselves, but that it's all only provisional and that one day, real life will begin. We prepare for death complaining that we have never lived. Sometimes I'm haunted by the thought that we have only one life and that we live it provisionally, waiting in vain for the day when real life will begin. And so life passes by . . .

— Ignazio Silone, *Bread & Wine*

Isn't it heartbreaking to consider how many of us have already lived so much of our lives provisionally, waiting, as Silone says, for the day when real life will begin? It is astonishing to consider how often we have compromised in the face of threats to our values and to ourselves. Why are so many of us lacking the courage to truly live the one life we have?

David Whyte tells the story of a friend of his who is asked to support an idea of his boss's. His boss wants him to say the idea is a "10." David's friend thinks it's not a very good idea and yet he hears himself say to his boss, in a mousy voice, "Yes, it's a 10, sir." Each time we surrender like this, some part of our soul breaks off and floats away. Yet these pieces of our broken souls can be retrieved. What it takes is courage and a commitment to purpose. We need to begin living our lives and living out what we believe — in our work each day.

In my companion book to this work, I discuss at length the practices that form the foundation for loving leadership. These practices arise from the central notion that the key motivating element for healing leaders is not money or power or fear, but meaningful purpose.

Victor Frankl, in his book *Man's Search for Meaning*, credits a clear sense of purpose for giving him the strength to survive three years in a concen-

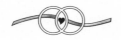

tration camp. Of equal import are his comments on the degree to which the absence of a sense of purpose resulted in the deaths of some inmates. Some, he says, died within twenty-four hours of uttering three devastating words: I give up.

Perhaps the best illustrations I've heard of the acute impact of purpose in generating energy are the stories that come from sudden emergencies. These are the frequently reported stories of young mothers who actually find the strength to pick up full-sized automobiles all by themselves. What is the motivating purpose? Their small children are trapped under the cars. Clearly, they would be unable to lift these cars absent the energizing goal of freeing their children.

Some of the best leadership lessons that have appeared in recent film literature are the great stories in the first three Star Wars films. These lessons are strong in large part because of the counsel of the late, great Joseph Campbell, who advised George Lucas and the screenwriters of these films. In one sequence from *Return of the Jedi*, the young apprentice, Luke Skywalker, tells the ancient Jedi Master, Yoda, that he will try to accomplish a certain hard task. Yoda responds. "Don't try . . . do . . . or do not," Yoda says, and in these words he instructs us on the pathway we must take to achieve the blessed environment of radical loving care. We must not be content with just trying. Leaders must do. They must make the hard decisions required to put in place a loving culture and they must persist in nurturing this culture when it has been developed.

It is undeniable that purpose and goal-setting are integral to success in our work lives — as well as in our personal lives. There is not space here for a detailed discussion of the Seven Practices of High Purpose Leadership. But I can list them for you and encourage you to read further about them in the companion book. I also encourage you to reflect on each of these practices for what the words may mean to you without any great amplification by me. Here is a very brief description of the practices:

1. Personal Commitment. Success is grounded on our clear and personal commitment to the highest possible purposes in our lives. When we consider our careers, we need to ask ourselves: Are we giving ourselves fully to our work? If we are not, why is this? Is it because we are in the wrong work? Is it because we are afraid? Or is it because we have never really made a conscious decision to commit to this work? Radical Loving Care requires that caregivers give themselves as completely as possible to their work because

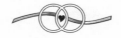

that is the only way patients will consistently receive healing care.

2. The Practice of Passion. After we have made a personal commitment to our work, we need to live out this commitment with passion. Half-hearted living does not reflect much of a commitment, does it? Passionate living means, first and foremost, that we discover how to fall in love with our work. Passionate baseball players, for example, love the game that they play. They love the baseball and the bat and the baseball diamond and the whole experience that goes with playing the game well. We need to cultivate this same kind of passion in our work — to love the people with whom we work and to love the place we work as well. This can be a hard exercise for someone who has never been passionate about anything. It can also be a wonderful awakening.

3. The Exploration of Potential. It is commonly believed that we live out only a small percentage of our true potential. This is very good news because it suggests that, if we are willing to challenge ourselves more, we can release some of our unused potential. The first question, however, must be for us to ask whether we are in the right work. There is no use struggling to release potential if we are in the wrong job. But once we have decided we are in the right work, the remaining task is to determine ways to unleash the enormous strength within us. The late Norman Cousins often said, "We are so much stronger than we think we are." He was right.

4. The Practice of Presence. This subject has been mentioned extensively elsewhere in this work. I raise it again here to advocate that you explore it in your development as a leader. Perhaps the single most important element of Radical Loving Care has to do with presence, because it is through true presence that we discover how to give our love to meet the needs of another. Presence requires that we work our way out of our own needs so that we may hear the needs of another — and that we then move to meet those needs.

5. The Practice of Positive Attitudes. Bob Hope said once, "Failure is the only thing I've been a success at."[60] We always hear that failure is the best teacher, but who's listening? And who wants to volunteer for a failure? Norman Vincent Peale was the best-known modern exponent of the concept of positive thinking. He knew that positive attitudes don't require that we sugarcoat everything and walk around with fake smiles pasted to our

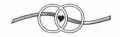

faces. Positive attitudes are important because of the energy they create for ourselves and for others. Positive attitudes create hope — and hope lives near the center of Radical Loving Care.

6. Persistence. This practice is akin to the expression of courage. Rollo May has written brilliantly about this subject: "Courage is not a virtue of value among other personal values like love or fidelity. It is the foundation that underlies and gives reality to all other virtues and personal values. Without courage our love pales into mere dependency. Without courage our fidelity becomes conformism."[61] There is nothing more important than persistence in the implementation of a Healing Hospital. There are so many setbacks that are certain to occur in the implementation of any new idea. If it's a truly worthwhile idea, like the Healing Hospital, then resistance is bound to be significant and persistence will be essential. Persistence is the power that causes us to hang in there even when we may, momentarily, have forgotten the reason that we should.

7. The Practice of Prayer and Meditation. A critical element of our journey to creating the Healing Hospital and to living out our own best vision is that we find ways to listen quietly for the voice of God. Regular practice of prayer or meditation or both is the reflective way through which we may sense whether we have aligned our work with God's love. Prayer and/or meditation are also an essential ingredient of self-healing. When we are engaged constantly in the world of action and ideas and never reserve time for balanced reflection, we experience wounds. Without the calming influence of reflection, we may be more inclined to wound others as well. This fact reinforces the importance of reflection as essential to healing work.

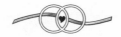

Chapter 6

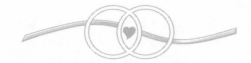

CARE PARTNERS™, CARE CIRCLES™, AND INTEGRATIVE MEDICINE

CHANGE THROUGH CARE PARTNERS: A KEY PROGRAM[60]

Care Partners are a small band of carefully selected employee partners who focus on special care for patients sixty-five and older. Their work is augmented by Care Companions, who are a mixture of volunteers and employees who sit with older patients who have special needs. Care Partners are available to senior patients twenty-four hours a day. Under the leadership of Perri Lynn White, their work at Baptist has not only resulted in better care for the senior population but has resulted in a reduction in patient falls.

When I first offered this idea at Baptist in late 1999 and early 2000, I could feel the skepticism. The nursing department leadership, who eventually embraced the idea, first felt somewhat protective of the status quo. They were concened that a new group of partners might encroach on the caregiving role of nurses. Ultimately, it became clear that Care Partners were greatly enhancing care and were actually freeing nurses to do other critical work.

The impact of Care Partners is often hard to measure precisely, but we know that it is powerful in the lives of some by their testimonials. One way to gauge their impact is to ask the ultimately human question: If your aged mother or father needed to be hospitalized, would you feel better or worse if they had a loving care partner available to them twenty-four hours a day? In a loving sense, every old person is our mother or our father. Especially in times of illness, we owe them the service that Care Partners are uniquely capable of providing.

There is a related question at a logical level: Are elderly patients more or less likely to fall if a Care Partner or Care Companion is present? Doesn't wisdom tell us that our senior population is deserving of special support and that the small cost of a Care Partner program is an excellent answer?

The development of the Care Partner program is a classic example of an idea that flows from the thinking that is typical in a Healing Hospital. Loving intention tells us every hospital should have a program like this. All we have to ask ourselves is this: "How would we like our mothers and fathers and grandparents to be treated?" Clearly, the Care Partner/Care Companion program 1) increases patient satisfaction, 2) relieves pressure on other caregivers, including nursing staff, and 3) is likely to reduce the incidence of patient falls.[62]

CHANGE THROUGH CARE CIRCLES: A KEY PROGRAM TO SUPPORT THE SERVANT'S HEART

Or could we change at last and choose truth?

— Robinson Jeffers

Telling the truth is hard in corporate life. The press of organizational politics encourages partners to compromise and play loose with the truth for fear of offending another partner or, God forbid, the boss. Putting up false fronts and pretending to like things we don't can be exhausting. In fact, professionals are constantly being asked to do this. We need to offer a sanctuary to our staff members. A place where they can speak freely and unburden their hearts. A place where we can choose truth.

The concept of implanting vision and expanding beliefs through small groups is at least as old as the Christian disciples in the first century. Small groups are places where healing is found, relationships are developed, understanding is advanced, and, typically, commitment rises.

Most organizations may feel they don't need a small-group approach. If you work in an organization like that, it may suggest there is very little passion around the vision of the organization. Can you imagine the growth of the Christian church without discipleship through small groups? Can you

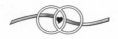

picture the advancement of the civil rights movement of the 1960s without the church network that Martin Luther King, Jr., used so effectively?

Organizations work in teams. In a Healing Hospital, team members need to meet in Care Circles. These can be established by assignment. Here's how they work:

1. Partners meet periodically (once a week or once a month) in their Care Circle for at least one hour.
2. The Care Circle may be made up of partners from different parts of the organization. An ideal size is anywhere from eight to twelve members.
3. Each group needs a trained facilitator.
4. The agenda for the meetings is simple:
    a. Each meeting begins with an announcement of a topic connected to the Healing Hospital — for example, "What does it mean to have a Servant's Heart?"
    b. Each member checks around the circle and shares with the group something about her or his work life and home life. The goal is sharing.
    c. As the group checks in, each person also offers comments on the topic of the day.
    d. Confidentiality is observed in order to encourage trust.
    e. People come to speak, share, and be heard — and also to listen. But it is not a problem-solving group. Other members do not criticize or offer advice.

Experiments with this approach at both the Fetzer Institute and at Baptist Hospital suggest that there are several helpful outcomes:

1. Members develop better skills at listening to each other and at practicing presence.
2. Participants feel a deeper commitment to each other and to the organization.
3. Participants are less likely to experience burnout since the group can provide a better sense of meaning and of belonging.
4. Mission and vision are better understood, and partners improve their ability to advance the vision in the rest of their work.
5. Productivity increases are likely.

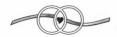

There are also hazards:

1. The circle process depends on trust and this can lead to vulnerability. Without effective facilitation, there is always a risk of hurt feelings.
2. Many staff will likely be skeptical at the beginning of this approach because the circles are not about *doing* something but about *being* someone.
3. The approach is most likely effective with salaried staff since hourly staff would need to use part of their shift or be paid overtime.

The Caring Circles approach is strongly recommended as a key way to advance mission in a Healing Hospital. It is also a superb way to advance the power of storytelling. The right stories are pivotal in a Healing Hospital. The stories are already there: the need is to find them and tell them. These stories, like the story of the housekeeper and the old man, signal the values of the organization.

THE ROLE OF INTEGRATIVE MEDICINE

The so-called integrative medicine movement in America is important. I first heard this phrase from the lips of Andrew Weil, M.D., a now well-known Harvard-trained physician who advocates balance in medical care between the learning of the west and the wisdom of the east.

In fact, wisdom tells us that many eastern-based medical treatments, including acupuncture, aromatherapy, massage, the use of certain herbs, and meditation seem to have a healing effect on many people. For example, the Chinese have demonstrated conclusively that some patients can be successfully anesthetized using only acupuncture and no drugs.

Still, because these approaches are primarily outcome-based rather than evidence-based, western medicine has been noticeably recalcitrant about allowing them into hospitals. This refusal is tragic and has blocked countless patients from the benefits of properly applied complementary therapies as an adjunct to western medicine.

Some of the more enlightened American healthcare organizations have sponsored limited use of complementary medicine under hospital auspices, including Harvard Medical School with its support of the work of Dr. Herbert Benson on the stress-reducing effects of meditation. Other enlightened work has come from Dr. Dean Ornish, with his outstanding

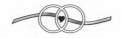

exploration of the impact of low-fat diets, meditation, and exercise as a therapy to treat heart disease. In addition, many hospitals, including Baptist in Nashville, have allowed the practice of acupuncture by M.D.'s in clinic settings.

Unfortunately, insurance companies still generally refuse to cover payments for these treatments. This makes economic viability problematic. Yet integrative medicine needs to be woven into the fabric of a Healing Hospital because 1) it frequently generates improved patient outcomes, 2) it makes sense, 3) it is minimally invasive, and 4) contrary to western medicine, eastern therapies rarely cause negative outcomes. In other words, the first axiom of the Hippocratic oath, not to do harm, is honored more successfully by complementary therapies than it is by traditional western medical approaches.

Healing Hospitals need to include integrative medicine in their care models. These therapies have been kept away from patients for too long. In the hands of the proper practitioners, integrative medicine can be more healing for patients than the use of traditional medical treatments by themselves.

PRESENCE TRAINING

We have spent so much time and effort teaching caregivers to be distant, clinical, and removed in their care that it now requires active training to teach partners and doctors how to reconnect with patients in a meaningful way. We have been taught to struggle to find an answer outside of us, not to look within — to wait and be present. Elizabeth Krueger, M.D., says, "It's taken me years to undo the damage of my medical training — and I haven't yet." She seeks to be present to her tiny patients and their parents. To do this she has to fight against physician training that tells her to keep her distance.

Our caregivers have been given the message that if you get too close to patients a couple of bad things will happen: 1) you'll lose focus and 2) too much emotional involvement will cause "burnout." The partial truth inside this rationale has caused a harmful disconnect in patient care. It has caused countless caregivers to interpret distance as meaning cold detachment. Certainly, patient relationships must be appropriate, but it turns out that meaningful presence to patient needs does not cause either loss of focus or burnout. Instead, it improves care and causes caregivers to discover that their work is meaningful.

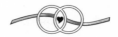

Tracy Wimberly initiated presence training at Baptist Hospital during 2000 and 2001. The training included a one-day program to help caregivers practice getting back in touch, including a range of exercises focused in part on introspection. Relationship-building was also practiced in groups of fifteen to twenty partners at a time.

This work needs to be part of every Healing Hospital. I have underestimated its importance in the past. Now I understand, after three decades of hospital leadership, that this training is essential because it is the single best way for staff members to practice each and every element necessary to create a Healing Hospital.

Presence training involves inviting a team into a room and giving them a full day to practice "presence exercises." These exercises can begin with a period of silent meditation in which each person is asked to reflect on the ways they can be present to another. I believe that an effective way to follow up is through exercises like the following:

1. **Importance of Presence.** Ask the group to discuss why presence is important in a caregiving setting. Encourage the citing of examples in which presence demonstrated the respect and valuing of another person.

2. **Painting/Music exercise.** Hold up a copy of a famous painting in front of the group. Ask them to look at the painting for one full minute. After this, ask what each of them sees in the painting. Then ask them to look again for one more minute and play some kind of music during this minute. This time, ask people to share what they felt while looking at the painting. The facilitator should receive each response without judgment.

3. **Pairings exercise.** Pair people up. Ask one member to take three minutes to share a problem of some kind with the other person. The listening partner is asked to demonstrate full presence during the three minutes. Then the partners switch. At the end of the exercise, ask the group a) to share what was difficult about staying present to the other person, b) how they think they could be present more effectively, and c) what they appreciated most in the listening of the other person.

4. **Repeat** the above exercise, but this time, the assignment is a medical simulation. Ask two partners to perform this simulation in front of the rest of the group. One partner is assigned the diagnosis of a stroke that has made him or her unable to speak,

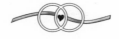

while the other person is assigned to be a caregiver. Ask the group to comment on the way these individuals are present to each other.

5. **Presence models.** Ask the group to share examples of people who are truly present to them in their lives and what effect this has on them. Discuss techniques people used to help them be present. Discuss the challenges to presence.

6. **Field exercise.** If the course is being taught in a hospital, send everyone out onto the floors for one hour and ask them to observe illustrations of presence that they see. They should take notes, asking themselves along the way about the impact of presence on caregivers and on patients.

These are just examples of some of the things that raise awareness of presence. You can build on these in any way you think appropriate. The key is to highlight the importance of this critical skill so that partners can learn how to integrate presence skills into their lives.

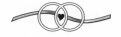

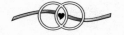

Chapter 7

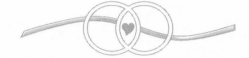

SUSTAINING THE
SERVANT'S HEART

*For this is wrong, if anything is wrong: not to enlarge the freedom
of a love with all the inner freedom one can summon. We need,
in love, to practice only this: letting each other go. For holding
on comes easily; we do not need to learn it.*

— Rainier Maria Rilke

One of the toxic characteristics of command/control leadership is its tendency to crush the freedom of others. Leaders who use this style tend to be chronically distrustful of everyone. They have an obsessive need to control their employees as if they owned them and could manage their every action. As Rilke says, "holding on comes easily; we do not need to learn it." What we need to learn is to love others enough to trust them and to let them go. This means appealing to what Lincoln called "the better angels" of the nature of others and trusting them to use their best instincts in advancing loving service.

Most people seem to know what it means to have a Servant's Heart. They know that it's about serving others. As Deschelle, a housekeeper on staff at Baptist, tells me, it's about "serving other people no matter what."

We may know the words, but the number of people who *live out* the call-ing of the servant in their work is fairly small. This small group can be greatly increased!

THE AUTHENTIC SERVANT'S HEART

One of the challenges of genuine service is that it asks that we try not to impose on others what *we* want, but what *they* need. Servant leaders seek to understand how to meet the needs of their staff. They also act with authentic intention to serve rather than from an ulterior personal motive.

One of the reasons compassion is difficult is that it requires that we enter into the pain of another. As Nouwen says, "…wanting to alleviate pain without sharing it is like wanting to save a child from a burning house without the risk of being hurt." This work can be exhausting, so caregivers often feel they need to protect themselves.

Just today at lunch, I asked a doctor how she went about giving lov-ing care in her practice of internal medicine. "I'm an actress," she said. "I have to pretend to be compassionate. If I actually tried to be genuinely compassionate to each patient, I would be completely exhausted by noon."

But does this have to be true? Aren't there ways for us to share the pain of another without collapsing? Some people have found successful solu-tions. Most often, they have learned to give themselves ways to rest and heal across the day.

The source of the true Servant's Heart is mysterious. Why is it that some people are almost natural servants while others seem to find it diffi-cult to lift a finger on behalf of another? It is useful for us to acquire an understanding of this because of how it helps us in two ways. First, an understanding of a servant may help us select those who will be our best partners. Second, if leaders understand the Servant's Heart better, they may know better how to support the periodic healing that a servant needs in order to sustain loving service.

As usual, it may be helpful to look at famous examples since they are widely known (although the fact that some servants are famous should not blind us to the fact that there are remarkable servants around us all the time). Mother Teresa was a person who faced straight into the most har-rowing pain of others. Across the day, she found relief in the quiet space of periodic prayer. But the key to Mother Teresa's remarkable vigor was that she was engaged in work she found meaningful. As David Whyte has

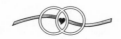

written, "a life that honors the soul seems to have a kind of radical simplicity at the center of it."[63] And a certain simple clarity about our life's calling and our work's meaning is the best source of vitality for all of us. With meaning there is hope. That is why it is so critical that servant leaders help frontline staff members understand why their work is sacred or meaningful. Hope and positive feelings are the motivators that create a productive workforce that truly wants the organization to succeed because it is their organization.

Many companies have taken this point literally. They have created employee-owned organizations. But this is a form of physical ownership and does not automatically generate emotional commitment. In my experience with a stock company, employee ownership and stock options did not generate a *real* sense of ownership in many of the employees. Real ownership is more a spiritual matter than it is a money matter. Employees' sense of true ownership of a company is primarily a function of: 1) whether they believe in what the company is doing, 2) whether they love their work and work environment, and 3) how they are treated by their supervisors.

We are not all called to be a Mother Teresa. Yet we can find passion in our work and we can all find ways to improve our work atmosphere. We can support the creation of "quality of work life" areas, as Tracy Wimberly did at Riverside Methodist Hospital in Columbus. And leaders can be sure that the work atmosphere allows for both humor and times of meditation or prayer.

The Care Circles provide an ongoing opportunity to practice relationship-centered care with each other. And we need to be careful about personal intensity and the maintenance of balance. Senator Bobby Kennedy's answer to this issue was that we should always take our work seriously, but not ourselves. As the shining example of Southwest Airlines has proved over and over again, it is possible for employees to joke around in the midst of the serious work of flying airplanes — and to be enormously successful. For caregivers, lightheartedness is a great salve to the exhaustion that can come from compassionate care.

Ultimately, the source of the Servant's Heart may be mysterious, but its expression is clear and visible to any leader who is watching. And any leader interested in creating a culture of healing must be especially vigilant and proactive in searching out these special servants and supporting them in any way possible. These servants are the true heroes of caregiving, and their gifts must be celebrated now as never before.

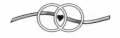

EMPLOYEE BENEFITS

There is an intensely practical side to all this, and it has to do with the apparently black-and-white world of employee benefits. Of course anyone who has spent any time in this complex area knows it is colored in subtle layers of gray rather than stark black or white. In my judgment, the key to a successful employee benefits plan doesn't lie in the specific *amount* of either pay or benefits. So long as pay and benefits are reasonably competitive, the question becomes not how *much*, but how *creatively and effectively* the benefits will meet employees' needs. It is important to follow a simple guiding principle presented as two questions: 1) what are benefits that really make a difference in partners' lives? and 2) can we provide these benefits cost-effectively?

In my work with Mark Evans, Tracy Wimberly, and Nancy Schlicting at Riverside Methodist Hospital, we achieved enormous success by thinking creatively. Here are four quick examples.

1. Day Care

Hospitals continue to be staffed predominantly by women. Even today, the bulk of the childcare responsibility falls in the lap of the mother. At Riverside, we didn't want our nurses (97% female) worrying a lot about the quality and reliability of daycare services. So we built a beautiful daycare center right in the middle of our parking lot and made sure it was staffed with first-rate teachers. The design was so creative that it included a tiny door at the entrance to the building just for small children to walk through. This effort was enormously successful for several reasons: 1) the day care was visible to all employees as a symbol of employer commitment, 2) parent/partners were pleased with both the quality of the facility and the quality of the teaching, which further signaled to employees that we valued them as family members as well as employees, and 3) the convenience was unbeatable and contributed, we believe, to positive employee morale.

2. Employee Convenience Center

At Riverside, an employee convenience center was established in cooperation with area merchants. It was set up in the middle of the parking lot of a one-thousand-bed hospital. Through this center, employees could place orders for groceries through a branch of Kroger food stores and pick up their order at the end of the day. The same was true with things like dry

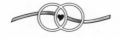

cleaning, shoe repair, and video rental. This was immensely popular and remarkably inexpensive. My recollection is that it cost the hospital less than $75,000 per year.

3. Employee Partner Recognition

It's always possible to have mechanical employee recognition ceremonies where service awards are handed out in assembly-line fashion, but with a little more creativity, these programs can become preeminent opportunities to celebrate the work of caregivers. At Riverside, with the special energy of one employee partner named Marcy Alton, these annual events were turned into lovely extravaganzas. An underappreciated dinner from the past was replaced with an hour-long program of recognition followed by the appearance of a name entertainer. This was accomplished by holding and videotaping smaller recognition ceremonies in advance, then showing the videos during the hour-long celebration. Employee partners felt honored in two ways: first by their special recognition on stage at the Ohio Theater and second through the presence of a big-name entertainer hired just to entertain the staff.

4. Leaders Working on the Front Lines

During most of the twelve years I led Riverside and the OhioHealth System, I would take one day a month to work a shift on the front lines in a different department. This is not something that can be done unless it is done with sincerity and is something a leader is willing to sustain over time. I did not require this of every leader, only those who really felt they could do it effectively. Frontline partners have an acute sense for phony behavior and that is why sincerity is so critical. In any case, this effort seemed to work extremely well — especially when the staff could see that I and other leaders weren't just playing around but were actually working through an entire shift.

Results!

The purpose of all these programs is to live out the philosophy that the main role of a hospital leader is to take care of the people who take care of people. Meanwhile, during this period the organization experienced: a) an extraordinary increase in productivity, b) a steady drop in turnover, c) a strong, significant, and sustained increase in bottom-line performance for *twelve straight years*, d) high patient satisfaction scores, and e) recognition on several top hospital lists — including listings as one of the best places to

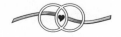

work in *Working Mother Magazine*, on an ABC television news special, and in the book *Service America*.

PRACTICING LOVING CARE

There is one more point about the Servant's Heart that needs to be emphasized. There is a mindset about loving care that requires regular practice. Giving love is not about us, it is about the recipient. A servant leader will constantly be thinking: "What are the kinds of things I can do to help the frontline staff?" A practitioner of Radical Loving Care would always be thinking things like: "My presence to a dying patient is about the quality of their final moments on this earth, not mine," and "If I hold the hand of a person in pain, it is to relieve their pain. It is not about me."

Ultimately, to expect that loving service can be delivered without some personal pain and fatigue is unrealistic. The truest answer is that compassionate care is both hard and important work. The best reward will always come from knowing how completely meaningful this kind of work is.

Henri Nouwen says that "the first and most important aspect of all healing is an interested effort to know the patients fully, in all their joys and pains, pleasures and sorrows . . . which have led them to their present situation."[64] And he says that "healing means, first of all, the creation of an empty but friendly space where those who suffer can tell their story to someone who can listen with real attention."[65]

Unfortunately for the beleaguered internist mentioned above, acting really doesn't work. Compassion requires genuine presence.

THE SERVANT'S HEART IN ACTION

We need to be a blessing to give a blessing.

— Deadre Hall, R.N.

I have met many true servants and have seen them at work. Remember Deadre Hall, R.N., the critical care nurse in the Neuro-Intensive Care Unit at Baptist in Nashville? She has gone through approximately the same ritual every morning for twenty-five years to prepare herself for the hard work she does each day. She says she asks God to bless her so that she can be a blessing for others. She also acknowledges something that every servant recognizes. She says, "I'm not perfect, I have my bad days, that's why I'm always asking God for help." As any of Deadre's patients can testify, she is

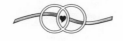

clearly a recipient of God's help because she is always passing her love along to others.

Lorraine Eaton, R.N., is another example. Lorraine's goal each day is to help her patients get through the hard experience in Intensive Care Units at Baptist so that they may hopefully recover and go home. "Refresh others and you will be refreshed," is a mantra that Lorraine repeats often to herself. She knows that most patients, because of the trauma of their conditions, will never remember her. Yet she gives her loving care to them each and every day.

To have a Servant's Heart means to commit to serve others above self. In order to be successful in building a Healing Hospital, it is critical to hire, orient, promote, and fire with this crucial quality in mind.

FOUR STEPS TO FILLING THE HOSPITAL WITH SERVANT'S HEARTS

Creating a positive employee environment begins with respect . . . It is really about respect and caring — qualities that motivate and energize people who are carrying out very difficult jobs 24/7/365.

— Nancy Schlicting, President and CEO, Henry Ford Health System

Step One: Hiring

The goal is to hire those candidates who either clearly possess a Servant's Heart or have the potential to develop this characteristic.

Who are these people and how do we find them? A key tool is what is generally referred to as "behavior-based interviewing." This is a fancy phrase for the kind of interviewing that focuses on more than just the résumé. This is interviewing that notices the commitment of the interviewee to his or her work. People who come to an interview expressing an obsessive interest in questions of pay and benefits only are those we try to avoid hiring in a Healing Hospital. Those who profess a genuine interest in caring for others and who demonstrate this in their background are the people we seek. Of course it is possible to fake it during the process. Still, good interviewers are perceptive and can separate the gold from the Fool's Gold.

Leaders should make clear to all staff members how important it is to hire for a Servant's Heart. It should be obvious that the interviewers themselves must have this characteristic. The very future of a Healing Hospital depends on an organization's success in hiring people who have the poten-

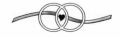

tial to commit deeply to the vision of the organization.

This whole issue is greatly underestimated. It is astonishing how much attention the traditional human resources department typically pays to educational credentials and how little attention is paid to attitude and outlook. Just because these things are difficult to quantify does not mean they are not important. Organizations that take hiring seriously find that they begin to have lower and lower turnover.

Step Two: Orientation and the IIF Formula

In late October, 1998, I spoke at my first orientation as the brand-new president of Baptist Hospital. I looked out expectantly at about fifty new employees. The first thing I saw were three employees in the back row — fast asleep! Several others looked close to sleep. Frankly, I couldn't blame them. The typical orientation program is almost as soporific as a PBS pledge break.

Nearly 75 percent of the Baptist orientation program at the time was presented with videotapes. This might not have been fatal if the videos had been good ones. Orientation is so boring in most hospitals that it is surprising that most people don't quit on the first day! In fact, most staff are so accustomed to monotonous orientations that it is the norm to assume they are just a necessary evil instead of a golden opportunity. We cannot hire for a Servant's Heart and then orient people as if they were robots! Orientation must be interactive, vital, and alive.

The good news is that orientation is one of the easiest things to change. The bad news is that if you only change orientation, you will create big disappointment when your partners leave orientation and arrive at their real jobs. The whole chain needs changing, and orientation is Step Two in the chain. What is needed first and foremost is the right attention from the right group of people.

> *We cannot hire for a Servant's Heart and then orient people as if they were robots!*

The central concept of good orientations is to build them on a three-part base, not the single pole on which they currently teeter. Bad (typical) orientations, like bad schoolteaching, rely exclusively on the attempted force-feeding of information. Of course the information never gets through to most of the audience. Good orientations emphasize what we call the *IIF formula: Information, Inspiration, and Fun.*

For the fun part, one might look at the incredibly successful orientation program at Southwest Airlines. Among other things, their orientation is

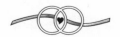

filled with joketelling and a lot of apparent "silliness." It is designed to create a warm environment for new staff. Accordingly, this organization is widely known for its consistently friendly staff. They are trained to integrate fun into their otherwise serious work — and consider how serious their work is. These people are involved in flying airplanes under strict government regulations. Yet they have one of the best safety records in the business. By the way, they also are typically number one in passenger satisfaction, employee morale, on-time departures, and profitability — even though they are a discount airline.

Southwest Airlines is a terrific example of the importance of hiring and orientation. What's baffling is that more organizations haven't successfully copied them!

Step Three: Regular Staff Reviews and the Firelight Window

> *I want to free what waits within me*
> *so that what no one has dared to wish for*
> *may for once spring clear*
> *without my contriving.*
>
> — Rainer Maria Rilke

I believe deeply that we all yearn to free what waits within us — to celebrate our life in our work. The most eloquent work I have read on this subject is the brilliant writing of David Whyte, author of both *The Heart Aroused* and *Crossing the Unknown Sea*. Whyte, a poet himself, would agree that the most eloquent poetry comes from Rilke when he sings about wanting to "free what waits within me" and to do so "without my contriving." This is like the alignment of a tuning fork with the right note on the piano. When the right note is found there is an easy and beautiful resonance. Until then, all the wrong notes create dissonance. In this dissonance there is a natural struggle to find the matching note. All the dissonance dissolves when that one right note is found. And there is only one right note in all those keys on the piano.

We need to figure out how to line up with the right note — how to get out of the way so we can let God come through us. We want to express our passion in our work, but society and its systems may beat us down. We often withdraw the milk of human kindness and replace it with a sour mixture of cynicism that bespeaks deep fear.

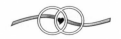

There are some who escape this cynicism. They are the ones we speak of here as having a Servant's Heart. They are not essentially different from other partners except that they have overcome their fears and decided to commit their best efforts to their work. We need to find methods of honoring these people and of helping others to either join them or to depart from the organization. The best tool for this, in a Healing Hospital, is the Firelight Window.

The Servant's Heart & The Firelight Window

Tool — The Firelight Window*

High Fire High Light	High Fire Low Light
Low Fire High Light	Low Fire Low Light

*The Firelight Window is adapted, in part, from a model developed in leadership training at General Electric Corporation on evaluating staff around results and values.

The Firelight Window is a tool of fundamental value in building a Healing Hospital. When it comes to hiring, orienting, reviewing, and firing, this window is a key guide. It has been used in a different form at General Electric, and it can help leaders in their regular efforts to both develop and review staff performance. We should be looking for strong performance (fire) as well as strong values (light).

I. Top Left Quadrant: Great Performance and Great Values (High Fire, High Light)

The core of a Healing Hospital emphasizes both performance outcomes and values. Ideally, a Healing Hospital is populated by staff members who balance great values with great performance. These are the partners who

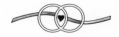

routinely demonstrate an ability to achieve excellent results with high integrity. These are the dream employees everyone wants to have. In a Healing Hospital, a conscious and sustained effort is made to support and retain these partners. In fact, when I have encountered partners in this category who threaten to leave for another job or retire, I usually pull out all the stops to try to retain them. Great employees attract other great employees, and their departure should never be taken lightly. In a Healing Hospital, the job may be replaceable, but *no person is replaceable* because each person is valued as unique.

II. Lower Left Quadrant: Kind but Ineffective
(Low Fire, High Light)

Partners in the lower left quadrant are characterized as people who have lovely values in general. They are the kind of people you would love to have as friends or dinner partners. The problem is that they *seem* to lack the fire to generate good results in their current role. It is quite likely that people in this quadrant may seem to lack fire because they are simply in the wrong position — and may be with the wrong organization. The goal in the improvement plan is to see if that fire can be awakened in their current role. If not, the kindest thing for all concerned is to attempt to guide these people toward settings where their passion may be ignited.

III. Top Right Quadrant: Effective, but Unkind or Unfair
(High Fire, Low Light)

We often see partners who achieve what appear to be strong results. On further examination we find they have gotten these results in spite of displaying poor values.

A classic example of this is the surgeon who is the owner of both talented hands and a terrible temper. Quite often during the past three decades a nurse has come to me with the complaint that a particular surgeon has lost his temper, shouted at the staff, and thrown his instruments. Over my years as a hospital CEO, when I would inquire further about constructive discipline in cases like this, the usual response would be something like: "Well, Joe has a bad temper, but he's a great doctor." In a Healing Hospital, *there is no such thing as a great doctor who treats others with disrespect.* Otherwise good doctors or nurses with anger problems need to be directed to anger management counseling..

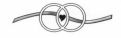

IV. Lower Right Quadrant: "Self-Firers" and "Radar Dodgers" (Low Fire, Low Light)

The lower right quadrant is made up of a group I typically refer to, somewhat flippantly perhaps, as "self-firing." What's unfortunate is how long many of these partners will hang around an organization. Some of them have developed a particular skill I call "radar dodging."

Every large organization seems to have a few of these — they are people who are both ineffective and not very well motivated, yet no one ever seems to get around to letting them go. They seem to have an instinct for how to fade into the woodwork whenever there's a layoff and will often outlast partners who are far more useful to the organization. Radar dodgers cannot dodge effectively in a Healing Hospital.

The key to dealing with partners in the top right or lower left quadrant of the Firelight Window is a pattern of three to six months of leadership counseling to attempt to move these partners over into the desired top left category. This counseling is done through a review process.

Review Process

If you don't walk the talk, no one will believe you or what you are trying to do.

— Elaine Ullian, President and CEO, Boston Medical Center

The goal is to review and evaluate each partner using the Firelight Window. This provides some sense of structure to a process that will always include significant subjectivity.

Until partners see that top leadership takes loving care and the Servant's Heart seriously, it will be difficult to move the culture in a hospital. On the other hand, leadership that truly chooses to commit to transforming hospital culture into an environment of healing, versus simply curing, can accomplish noticeable changes in as little as one year. The reason for this is that most caregivers are simply waiting for the support of leadership to release the loving power within them.

A useful way to consider how a culture can change is to remember the Wave Theory. Leaders don't have to convince one hundred percent of the staff in order to change the culture. In fact, culture change can often be accomplished by moving less than half the staff.

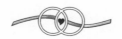

Step Four: Firing the Non-Servants and Clearing Out the Bullies

It is not how much we do, but how much love we put into doing it. It is not how much we give, but how much love we put into giving.

— Mother Teresa

In building a Healing Hospital, it is as important to rid the organization of non-productive and wrongheaded staff as it is to hire servants. This does not mean the elimination of opposition! In fact, every Healing Hospital needs loving critics who are prepared to point out deficiencies in the model and to constructively express an opposing point of view.

One of the ways I would always know things were headed in the right direction in the hospital was when I would hold a meeting with employee partners and a staff member would complain that they needed more support to serve patients better. This is a sign of a desire to serve more effectively, not a negative or destructive complaint.

In any case, there is an enormous difference between constructive opposition and destructive whining. The low-performance whiners who complain *to patients* about pay and staffing and also the mean tyrants who lead by intimidation both *need to be removed*, no matter how tight staffing is!

I always think, here, about the true story of the high school basketball coach portrayed in the movie *Hoosiers* who threw two of his best players off the team for arrogant behavior, leaving him with only five players. He knew the value of having the right team culture. His integrity, in that case, helped him build a team that came out of nowhere to win the 1954 Indiana High School Basketball Championship.

> *The low-performance whiners ... and the mean tyrants who lead by intimidation need to be removed, no matter how tight staffing is!*

Constructive critics are a great value in a Healing Hospital . . . and it is important to respect those who honestly support command/control leadership styles. That approach has its place, perhaps, but it is not the style of the Healing Hospital. Leaders who believe the only way to lead is by ordering their staff around will defeat the Healing Hospital model. They must be encouraged to seek work elsewhere or be fired in a respectful way.

Like you, I have encountered many bullies in my lifetime — both inside work settings and elsewhere in the world. I have a very low tolerance for bullies in any environment. Bullies prey on people they perceive

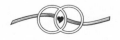

as weak or vulnerable. In the workplace, the bully is the tyrant leader who uses his or her leadership position to pick on or torment subordinates. Loving leadership requires the courage to remove tyrants.

It is remarkable how much tyrannical behavior exists in corporate America. Most large organizations contain a certain number of leaders who abuse their authority over others. At Baptist, I noticed some examples of this when I arrived, and I worked to eliminate that behavior and the individuals who practiced it. To act against tyrannical behavior is an essential part of positive leadership.

When bullies are allowed to run free in a work setting, it creates a terrible environment for the advancement of loving care. Abusive behavior can chill a work environment to the point where people are always afraid of being fired arbitrarily. This means that employee partners will also 1) tend not to offer any new ideas or creative thinking, 2) spend time blaming others, and 3) hold back on their best efforts because they resent the environment.

How do you advance loving care in an environment like this? Dictatorial and arbitrary leaders are not the ones to advance a mission of loving care. They must be rooted out and removed. Yet this is often difficult, and successful elimination of bullies requires both careful planning, skillful execution, and an approach that preserves respect and integrity.

The point is that the Healing Hospital model is incompatible with the intimidating style that characterizes most command/control managers. Bullies are a curse in any organization — but they are absolutely inimical to the success of a Healing Hospital.

COUNSELING AND FIRING

When working with partners who fall in either the top right or lower left quadrants of the Firelight Window, you can counsel them for three to six months along the lines of servant leadership (see the Seven Practices of High Purpose Leadership on pages 145–146). If there is no meaningful progress, then it's time to change these people out.

> *Love requires that we ... hold staff accountable.*

The justification for this is that it's not fair to subject staff or patients to the oppressive leadership of dictatorial leaders. Loving care simply cannot thrive under a dictatorship because dictatorship

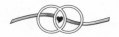

undermines the dignity and worth of other leaders.

Similarly, caregivers who insist on strictly cold, transactional encounters with patients must be provided with counseling. After a reasonable time, if they are unable to balance their technical work with kind-hearted care, they must be removed. Just as crucially, if a caregiver is kind-hearted but incompetent, clearly she or he must be put through the same process. It is *unloving* to subject patients to care that is either uncaring or incompetent. *Loving care calls out for clinical excellence.* Every review, training, and promotion process must incorporate the use of this Firelight Window approach. Although every model has flaws, this tool will bring strong results if applied effectively by enlightened leaders.

At the core of loving leadership is the fundamental notion of individual accountability. Love requires that we take responsibility and hold staff accountable for commitment to mission. To make a decision based on rules alone is not only foolish but promotes bureaucratic thinking. To make a decision based solely on personality or ego is damaging to organizational integrity. The goal must be to make decisions informed by mission and simple guiding principles.

LAYOFFS AND OTHER TERMINATIONS

One of the most horrifying mistakes that many healthcare leaders routinely make is the savage termination of capable and committed people. We all know those stories. These are the dedicated employees who have given ten or twenty or thirty years of their work lives in committed service to their employer. Suddenly one day they are rudely notified, via those infamous "pink slips," that they are either being laid off, or worse, permanently terminated.

The feeling of sudden, savage, and unjustified termination is often experienced like any other significant loss — like a death or like a diagnosis of cancer. I have even heard people refer to a sudden termination as causing them to feel as though they had been raped. It is almost incomprehensible how leaders who might otherwise consider themselves caring can inflict layoffs so thoughtlessly.

Please note that I am not questioning the need to sometimes terminate an otherwise capable person for, perhaps, financial reasons. The issue here has to do entirely with respect. I strongly disagree with the practice engaged in by some hospitals of laying off dedicated people with the use of security guards. I have heard of many examples of this and I think it's criminal-style

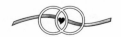

behavior. The practice is also a sure way to 1) destroy morale among the remaining staff, 2) instill permanent enmity in the people terminated like this, and 3) raise the risk of lawsuits.

On the occasions when I have terminated capable people due to financial reasons, I have done my best to be honest and respectful. This means giving the individual plenty of time to clear out their office, reasonable severance, outplacement services, and when the person wants it, a going-away party. It also means not offering phony explanations for the termination or engaging in defensive responses. In 1998, when I let some executives go at Baptist due to our huge losses, one of them told me he thought this was very unfair. I agreed with him. I said, essentially, "You're right, it is unfair to have to let a capable person like you go. You're a good man. We just don't have the money to pay you." He told me he appreciated my honesty and, to his credit, he continues to be a friend of the organization.

When a person has served an organization in a dedicated way and is being terminated for, say, a reorganization, why wouldn't the employer want to honor the individual for his or her years of dedicated work? This may include partners who have served well for short periods as well as long-term veterans. The issue is the quality and commitment of the partner's service. What is the signal sent to the rest of the staff when long-term partners suddenly disappear? Even worse, I have heard of cases where remaining employee partners are actually instructed not to communicate with a terminated staff member even when the staff member was an honored partner who was not terminated for cause. This is disrespectful and unwise. How would you feel if you were told you couldn't speak with someone you'd worked with for fifteen years who was terminated merely because of a reorganization? When employers fire dedicated people and those people suddenly vanish without a trace, there is deep harm done to the soul of the organization. In a Healing Hospital, dedicated partners must always be honored — especially when they are departing after years of valuable service.

FOUR KEYS FROM A
TOP HUMAN RESOURCES EXPERT

Mark Evans, the best Human Resources leader with whom I have worked, offers some key ways to create an employee-friendly hospital. Below, in his words, are four of his keys.

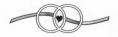

1. *Know why a positive work environment is important.*

When busy leaders are forced to prioritize, they must have a high level of commitment to devote the necessary time to create this kind of workplace. Leaders must believe in their hearts that creating a positive work environment is critical to success. This is not something they do to be nice or to be liked by their associates; while these are worthwhile objectives, they are not compelling enough to carry the day when hard decisions have to be made.

The connection between organizational success and employee satisfaction is easy to make, especially in a hospital. Anyone who has been a patient or tended to a family member in a hospital knows that how care is given is oftentimes as important as what care is given. Medical professionals can only have the best interactions with their patients if they feel good about the organization they are a part of and how they are treated there.

Leaders should continually seek to demonstrate to their staff leaders the correlation between employee satisfaction and high-quality patient care. Medical professionals are scientists and value studies that quantify relationships. Create studies that measure both sides and show the connection. Interview employees about how their feelings influence their work with patients and families, and report the results of these interviews.

2. *Ask employees what is important.*

If leaders want to know what they can do to increase the level of satisfaction in their areas of responsibility, they should begin by asking.

This asking should be done in many different ways to allow all employees to provide input regardless of their personal communication style. Some are more comfortable with written surveys, while others prefer a focus group setting. Some like one-on-one discussion with their supervisor, while others might like to provide written feedback. Managers learn a great deal by being present with the staff and asking very informally, "What can we do to make this a better place to work?" All these techniques and many more work to identify what employees think are important. Effective leaders are constantly dreaming up new creative ways to get feedback.

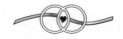

Many managers are reluctant to ask for this kind of input, fearing that it might make them look bad. The key is to adopt a continuous improvement mindset. It doesn't matter so much if the results are good or bad. What matters is that the leader is seeking input and will take positive steps based on the suggestions made. What matters is that in six months this will be a better place to work.

3. Develop specific programs to address the most common suggestions.

As leaders across the organization begin to seek ideas, they will identify patterns that cross departmental boundaries. Most commonly these relate to pay, benefits, opportunities for growth, training, etc. As these themes emerge, the top executives should recognize them and programs should be developed to address them. Frontline supervisors must carry enough influence that fixing the problems they identify becomes a high priority.

4. Recognize the importance of frontline supervisors.

Joe Vella was, for many years, the Vice President of Labor Relations for Federated Department Stores. Joe conducted training for managers who were expected to maintain a union-free workplace. He began the training with a presentation of research done by interviewing employees who had just voted in a union election.

Each person was asked how he or she had voted in the election and a series of questions regarding why. Very dramatically, Joe would ask the young managers in his class, "What is the #1 reason people voted for a union?" Invariably a hand would shoot up with the response: "Pay." Joe would tell them that pay was well down the list. Others would guess benefits or job security or physical workspace issues. "No, no, no . . . " Joe would tell them. "The number one reason people vote for a union is that they believe their immediate supervisor doesn't care about their problems, or they care but don't have the ability to do anything about them."

Joe Vella pointed out something I have observed over and over again. The most important person in the workplace is the employee's direct supervisor. A great, caring supervisor will make

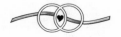

up for organizational problems. Poor supervisors will cause their associates to be unhappy even in a great organization.

Leaders working to create a more employee-friendly environment must focus on helping frontline supervisors. This includes a great deal of communication, training, and recognition.

SPECIAL CHALLENGE TO YOU

The challenge of the Servant's Heart is a challenge directly to you to choose now to write out the way that *you* would articulate your four keys. This exercise is critical because it will help you crystallize both what you value and how you would describe it to others. Do yourself and your organization a favor by doing this now and then returning frequently to your list to see how well you are doing in following up on what you believe.

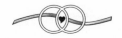

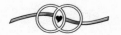

Chapter 8

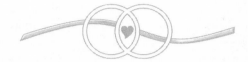

THE INTEGRAL ROLE
OF HUMOR AND PLAY

Question: *The Republican National Committee recently adopted a resolution saying you were pretty much of a failure. How do you feel about that?*

President Kennedy: *I assume it passed unanimously.*[66]

It's just ridiculous that I would wait until the end of this little book to talk about something everybody loves. I hope some of you have skipped ahead to read this part — or perhaps have looked at the table of contents to discover that this work is not just about work! Mark Twain's famous story of Tom Sawyer whitewashing the fence is one of the best examples I've ever read about how to integrate play into work. Yet it demonstrates even better how hard it is to get people to do menial work unless that work is thought of in an appealing way.

> *He can compress the most words into the smallest ideas better than any man I ever met*
> — Abraham Lincoln,
> referring to a lawyer.

I understand that studies have demonstrated that more Americans have heart attacks between 8 and 9 a.m. Monday morning than any other hour of the week. The second most frequent hour for heart attacks is just one hour earlier — between 7 and 8 a.m. on Mondays. We can see why this might be so. The American culture sends terrible signals about work. This starts with the signal that work and play are completely different and never the twain shall meet! There is a popular restaurant chain called TGIF's — (Thank God It's Friday's). Needless to say, there's no competing chain out there called TGIM's (Thank God It's Monday's). Maybe there should be! But what would they serve? Chicken noodle soup?

It doesn't need to be like this. We can celebrate our work by learning how to make it fun as well as challenging. At the beginning, we need to remember Robert Kennedy's words about taking our work seriously but not ourselves. There's nothing worse than the image of the self-important executive who struts down the hallway puffed up with his or her own importance.

The story is told about a previous leader at Baptist that he once called a doctor into his office to complain that the doctor had made jokes about the Dallas Cowboys — his favorite team. The doctor exclaimed that was just football talk. The next week, when the doctor was overheard to make more jokes about the Cowboys, the executive reportedly cancelled his contract to read electrocardiograms at the hospital. This kind of behavior not only suggests that the executive is taking himself far too seriously, but that any employee who tells a joke may be fired. The refusal to permit good-natured joking around can send a terrible chill through the culture of an organization.

> *Humor is powerful. But there is a misconception that people who use humor are less effective. This is not true...Studies show that people who use humor are 20% more productive.*
> — Mary Feeley, C.S.P

On the other hand, lightheartedness is thought to be one of the key reasons for the success of Southwest Airlines. Can you imagine the reaction of the more uptight personalities (if there are any) at Southwest when the suggestion was offered that jokes should be told during the reading of the FAA regulations to passengers? After all, the work of flying airplanes is deadly serious — but it turns out that this does not mean that the flight attendants have to take themselves so seriously. And as we all know, Southwest Airlines is one of the most successful in the country — and one of the safest.

What is the best way to integrate fun and humor into the workplace? First of all, the boss has to set the example. The safest humor is that which is always directed at the safest target for humor. To find this target, we need

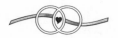

only look in the mirror.

I may not be the best example of this, but I can give you one illustration of how I attempted to use humor during my time at Baptist. You will recall that we were losing lots of money and things were pretty tense. I frequently included jokes at the beginning of my speeches and tried to signal the difference between the seriousness of the work and the need for lightheartedness otherwise.

As one way to signal lightheartedness, I used the issue of my rapidly thinning hair. We made a video that included a sequence of me talking to my staff about what a gigantic issue my hair loss was and how it could threaten the whole stability and credibility of the organization. On camera, I asked for their advice with mock sincerity — as if it were a matter of life and death. The video ended with a ridiculous scene in which the narrator reported that I had found the solution for my hair loss. I appear in the final frames in a huge wig. You're correct; you had to be there.

Sure, it's silliness. But what was accomplished with innocent nonsense like this was a strong signal to the one hundred fifty leaders who saw it that, hopefully, I didn't take myself too seriously. On the other hand, it's important that they already knew how sincere and passionate I was about our work together and how deeply I felt about the mission of our organization.

It's about the work; it's not about the boss. Whenever I've lost sight of this, it has meant I was making a mistake. I remember starting to take myself pretty seriously after I began hosting a television show that went into national syndication. It was called "Life Choices with Erie Chapman." The trouble began when I put my own name in the title. This sense of self-importance sometimes caused me to be too impatient with some of the staff, which is always counterproductive.

One thing that is just plain deadly to an organization or a country is a boss who can't tolerate jokes. We know this about former President Richard Nixon, who was notoriously self-conscious on the subject of humor. We also know that no dictator likes the idea of jokes and typically will display no sense of humor. Dictators want to be feared, and who's going to be afraid of a leader who makes jokes about him- or herself? It may be a sign you are in a toxic work environment if the boss forbids joking of any kind.

> *Mr. Nixon in the last seven days has called me an economic ignoramus, a Pied Piper, and all the rest. I've just confined myself to calling him a Republican, but he says that is getting low.*
> — John F. Kennedy

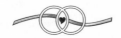

Of course certain kinds of joking can be inappropriate. But healthy joking creates a healthier work environment and can serve to relieve the stressful aspects of work. A great example of this occurred in a Super bowl game between the Cincinnati Bengals and the San Francisco 49rs. With less then a minute to go, the 49rs had the ball around midfield. With a touchdown they would win the game. What would you say to your team in the middle of this kind of tension? Thousands of fans were screaming and millions more were tuned in via television.

As I heard the story, Joe Montana came back to the huddle after a play. There were about forty seconds left in the game. He smiled, looked around at his teammates, and said, "Hey, you guys. Guess what, (comedian) John Candy is up in the stands!" According to players in the huddle, this little comment accomplished a few things: 1) it relieved the tension, 2) it signaled to everyone that the quarterback was relaxed and in control, and 3) it enabled the team to focus more effectively on the job at hand. Of course, the 49rs went on to score and win the Superbowl.

> *Politics is an astonishing profession. It has enabled me to go from being an obscure member of the junior varsity at Harvard to being an honorary member of the Football Hall of Fame.*
> — President John F. Kennedy

It's not required that every leader have the comic ability of Bob Hope or President John F. Kennedy. A sense of humor is a function of humility, not of brilliance. Humble people are able to see the humor in their own weaknesses. Humble leaders have the ability to balance all this with the strength needed to lead effectively. Humor is often the magic ingredient that restores balance in the midst of chaos.

Conclusion

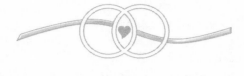

CONCLUSION

What are we afraid of, what stops us from speaking out and claiming the life we want for ourselves? Quite often it is a sudden horrific understanding of the intimate and extremely personal nature of the exploration.[67]

— David Whyte

What is it that can infuse our hearts with enough courage to face into the "personal nature of the exploration?" The courage to establish a Healing Hospital rises from a profound appreciation of the suffering that currently exists in America's hospitals. This suffering resides not only within patients but also within families. And it lives, as well, in the tired and discouraged hearts of millions of America's caregivers — and in some of their leaders as well.

Healing Hospitals seek to convert some of this suffering into joy by introducing love into all phases of leadership and all phases of clinical care. Currently, hospitals offer certain levels of disease treatment and pain relief. Healing Hospitals go far beyond this. The creation of a culture of loving service is aimed at convincing leaders that they need to truly take care of the people who take care of people. Frontline staff members who are treated with respect by leaders are significantly more likely to treat you and me with respect if we become patients.

Out of respect flows the opportunity for authentic loving service. A confused, sick old man calls out from his hospital room for his daughter. But his daughter has long ago left the hospital, and the housekeeper, who is mopping the floor outside his room, answers his cry instead. She takes his hand in hers. He quiets down. Soon he goes off to sleep. The housekeeper returns to the other part of her sacred work — cleaning the floor of a hospital. The loving housekeeper has picked up the ancient Golden Thread of healing and woven it into a Sacred Encounter. The love of a Servant's Heart has met the deep need of an old man.

So much depends upon our ability to appreciate that old man as our very own father or grandfather and to treat him with all the kindness with which we would like to be treated. We are all children of God. This means we are all brothers and sisters in this world. The screaming, stinking street person who wanders into the Emergency department bleeding is our brother. The four-hundred-pound woman who struggles in her wheelchair is our sister. The baby writhing with inherited cocaine withdrawal is our child — and his mother is our sister. And the man washing dishes in the kitchen of the hospital cafeteria is our brother as well.

In 1930, Albert Einstein wrote, "The most beautiful thing we can experience is the mysterious. It is the source of all true art and science." It is in the world beyond the grasp of either art or science where the greatest power abides. Indeed, art and science can barely reveal the outermost edge of this great mystery of God. As Michelangelo wrote, "The true work of art is but a shadow of the divine perfection." But as we pursue this shadow, we are gaining the best chance we have in this lifetime to touch the edge of the divine.

Two millennia ago, in the Sermon on the Mount, Jesus of Nazareth gave us the ultimate challenge for our life here on earth. He implored his listeners to put aside what they had heard before about an eye for an eye and a tooth for a tooth and hatred of one's enemies. Instead, he said, "Love your enemies and pray for those who persecute you." What a hard thing this is – and what a powerful test of our true belief in love. Jesus' radical statements about unconditional love are the foundation for the Healing Hospital concept. At the same time, the practice and expression of this loving service is clearly not aimed solely at Christian hospitals. Love is a universal concept, and humanitarian care is what every hospital must practice to be a place of true healing. Still, the message of Jesus about the need for each of us to love those who seem beyond love is critical for caregivers — especially those who are called upon to care for exceptionally difficult patients in extremely difficult circumstances.

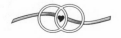

Above all, it is important that every hospital honor and observe the integrity of its own mission statement. We can no longer tolerate work environments that would punish a housekeeper for leaving her post to give loving service or settings that would ignore the cry of an old man. There is no need for us to keep repeating the mistakes of the past, or to cling slavishly to a status quo of mediocrity.

We can truly change all this — not in a week or in a year, but with a lifelong commitment to the missions by which we claim to live. We need to discover a new focus on giving loving care to others during the hard chapters of their lives on this earth. And that is the sacred opportunity before all caregivers and all healthcare leaders right now.

Now we have the opportunity to begin a whole new phase of our work in hospitals and other charities. Now is the time to restore hospitality to its rightful place. Now is the time for us to begin moving the wave toward the shore of loving care. Now is the time for us to emerge from the half-light of minimum effort and to abandon the gray land of sullen mediocrity that is strangling the love out of our hospitals and health clinics. We must create the kind of hospital setting that we would want for those we love — a Healing Hospital — where every single caregiver offers loving kindness to every patient and to each other. This is the kind of place where Radical Loving Care lives in a continuous chain of light. This is a possible dream, and with a meaningful commitment from enlightened leaders, this dream can become a reality.

I close as I began — with a challenge from my heart to yours in these words:

Be A Lover

The mystic chords of memory . . . will yet swell
when again touched by the better angels of our nature.
— Abraham Lincoln, March 4, 1861

> *Be a lover.*
> *All the disembodied voices*
> *of all your ancestors,*
> *are calling this to you now.*
>
> *Be a lover!*
> *Break free of the cold grasp*

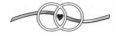

of all the things that sap
your life's best energy.

Drive away the dragons
of fear and restraint.

Climb into the arms of Lincoln's
better angels and

Be a lover.
All the voices
of all the saints
are calling this to you now.

I know the Siren's songs are calling too —
easy to hear and easier still to answer.
There are passions in you
and there was a Passion just for you.

So be a lover.
Not the one with lust
but the one with bread and wine who,
amid the dust
hears others' cries of thirst
and breaks the crust and brings
the living water just to nurse
the endless need.

There is an old man down the hall.
He calls to you. He has cancer.
You can hide or you can answer.

You can ride the wings
of angels and
be a lover.

— Erie Chapman, August 14, 2003

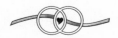

ACKNOWLEDGEMENTS

Love and appreciation are often difficult to express adequately. It would have been impossible for me to succeed in any aspect of my work without the love and support of my extraordinary wife, **Kirsten.** Her steadfast and caring presence across thirty-seven years of marriage and my multiple careers, her exquisite commitment to raising our two children, her eloquent writing, and her passionate attention to family and friends have taught me more about radical loving care than anything I have ever seen in a hospital.

My son **Tyler** has given me outstanding advice along the way about a number of issues that touch the work in this book. His wisdom is an ongoing inspiration to me. The photograph of the nurse caring for an elderly patient is emblematic of the fine photography of my daughter, **Tia.** She is a photographer because she has been wise enough to follow her passion and match it with one of her many gifts. Thanks to both of them for their love and support.

David Cox, M.Div., has provided invaluable service in the development and completion of this book. He has acted as editor, adviser, and reviser. I am particularly grateful to him for his willingness to listen patiently and wisely as I tried out endless ideas with him. His reflection, patience, and exceptionally intelligent insights have been invaluable in the creation of this work. I am also dedicated to poet, author, and speaker **David Whyte** for the inspiration his work has provided to me and to those of us who have developed the Healing Hospital. I strongly recommend his brilliant work to anyone who cares about restoring passion to America's workplaces. In addition, I would like to recognize **Jan Keeling** for her superb work in editing the second printing of this book.

Professor Bart Victor, Ph.D., of the Owen School of Management at Vanderbilt University, has been a very powerful influence on the direction this work has taken. His critique of the first several drafts of this book caused me to take a different direction on several key issues. His interest in my concept of magic and my subsequent concepts of Magi Theory caused me to zero in on this area for central focus in leadership training for the Healing Hospital. **Professor Douglas Meeks, Ph.D.,** of Vanderbilt Divinity School, read the earliest drafts of this work and helped to imbue in me a deeper understanding of the powerful role of stories in advancing vision and of the importance of focusing this work toward faith-based hospitals.

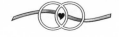

I would like to especially thank **Mr. Virgil Moore,** Chairman of the Board of the Baptist Healing Hospital Trust and the former Chairman of the Baptist Hospital System. His remarkably steadfast and caring leadership has been crucial to the success of both organizations. In addition, Mr. Moore is the best example of a true southern gentleman I have ever met. I am grateful for his ongoing commitment to advancing the ministry of loving service through the Healing Hospital concept. My thanks also to our other long-serving board officers, Vice Chairman **Ken Ross** and Secretary **Ed Moody** as well as **Dr. Bob Norman,** who is the funniest and most lovable preacher I ever met. Indeed, I am grateful to **all the members of the Board** for believing in this work and making it possible.

I would also like to thank my colleague **Stephanie Zembar, Esq.,** for her review of this work from a legal and financial perspective. Her skill enabled success in our work starting way back in Columbus and continued through Baptist Hospital and through today. The brilliant work of the extraordinary **Jeff Kaplan**, working with Stephanie and **Jim O'Keefe** and board member **Scott Jenkins,** enabled the successful sale of the Baptist Hospital system that generated the funds to support the Trust. Jeff is the most loyal and dedicated staff person with whom I have ever worked.

Special thanks to **Keith Hagan, M.D.,** for his dedicated and courageous leadership of the medical staff through the most difficult periods of transition at Baptist. It was a great blessing that he happened to be president of the medical staff at a crucial time in the development of the Healing Hospital. Dr. Hagan's sensitivity and well-developed spirituality are a continuing source of strength in the advancement of Radical Loving Care. Thanks also to former Chief Operating Officer **Dr. Paul Moore,** FACHE, for his sense of humor and his skills at affirming frontline staff members and physicians during the time I was president and CEO of Baptist Hospital System.

I appreciate the long-term guidance of my oldest and best friend, **Bill Banta, Esq.** Bill is the finest labor lawyer in the country and his wisdom about employee relations has guided companies coast to coast. Special thanks also for the patience and skill of **Bill Kersey** of KerseyGraphics who designed the text style and prepared this book for printing.

Kristin O'Keefe, Kristen Keely-Dinger, and **Michelle Polk** have also provided superb assistance in reviewing drafts of this book and ensuring that it reached successful completion. They have conscientiously studied paragraph after paragraph to ensure that the work was as error-free as possible.

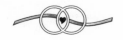

Thanks as well to **Dr. Richard Glenn and his team** at Saint Thomas Health Services for sharing their thoughts on the application of this work in the context of the hospitals they serve. Our ongoing partnership has enabled the work of the Healing Hospital to continue at Baptist and in the Saint Thomas system.

Kim Fielden, R.N., has been a key Healing Hospital leader during her time as Chief Nursing Officer at Baptist. **Debi Villines, R.N.,** is also a superb example of a loving person who continues her leadership at another hospital. Both of these women will do healing work wherever they serve. Baptist Hospital and its nursing staff were extremely fortunate to have Kim as Chief Nursing Officer and Debi as a director.

Tejuana Holmes, R.N.; Bubba McIntosh; Janet Keenan, R.N.; Holly Kunz, R.N.; Holly Smithey, R.N.; Karen Moore, R.N.; and **Perri Lynn White, R.N.,** are some of the superb leaders that are carrying out the clinical work of loving leadership in the Healing Hospital at Baptist and will do this into the future. **Jason Dinger** is one of the most capable young leaders I know. In addition, I would like to recognize **Cathy Self** for single-handedly picking up the teaching of the Seven Powers of High Purpose Leadership and teaching it to all new Baptist partners in orientation and also teaching it to countless other staff members. Her dedication to this work is both deeply touching and very effective. **Barbara Giannotti** has, along with Cathy, transformed orientation at Baptist and continues to refine it into one of the premier hospital orientation programs in the country.

One of the vehicles that brings the work of a Healing Hospital to light is extraordinary filmmaking. **Van Grafton** is the best videographer I've ever seen. He has been a wonderful partner working with me in the creation of the films *Sacred Work* and *The Servant's Heart.* Both of these films helped lay the groundwork for this book and this work. I am also deeply grateful to two additional dedicated people, **Darlene Hayes,** who served as my assistant from 1995 until the end of that decade, and **Rhonda Swanson,** who took over from Darlene. Darlene's dedicated support and listening ear were of endless help to me. Rhonda's help to me, both in my regular work and in my music composition, was transformational for my life. Her courageous battle with cancer is an example for anyone with a serious illness.

I am in the field of healthcare because of one man, the late **Bruce Trumm,** former President and CEO of Riverside Hospital in Toledo (now called Saint Ann). For reasons that remain mysterious, he called me one day out of the blue in 1975 to invite me to train to take his role at Riverside

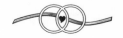

Hospital in Toledo. His generous spirit and large personality will always remain with me.

Bruce also introduced me to one of the most passionate caregivers I ever knew, **Marian Hamm, M.S.N.** Marian and I worked together across eight years in Toledo and then through the remarkable experience of Riverside Methodist in Columbus. In both places, she headed up patient care services. Her courage and incredibly skillful leadership transformed patient care at both Riversides. Her friendship and partnership transformed me.

A tiny number of us are fortunate to have the benefits of wise counsel from people who are actually professional counselors. I would like to publicly acknowledge the very private and confidential assistance of **Mary Lynne Musgrove.** Ms. Musgrove's counseling is rarely acknowledged because her communications are professionally privileged. I am pleased to thank her for her profound help across the past five years. She is a true spiritual being.

For twenty years, up through the middle of 2002 when she retired, my dear colleague and friend **Tracy Wimberly, R.N.,** worked side by side with me in the development of so much of this work. Her contributions endure at Riverside Methodist Hospital in Columbus through the ministry of the Hospice program she shepherded into existence and through several other programs such as the Elizabeth Blackwell Center. From 1983 through 1995, long before the name Healing Hospital was conceived, Tracy and our leadership team at Riverside Methodist and OhioHealth helped ensure that we had the same concepts in place in that organization that we subsequently developed at Baptist in Nashville. The thousands of employees who work in that organization will never know the debt they owe to Tracy for the quality of work life they enjoy today in that organization — the foundation for which was laid in the late 1980s. I will always be grateful to Tracy for her brilliant work.

Brilliance is also the word I would use to describe the groundbreaking work of **Mark Evans,** who is the finest Human Resources Executive I ever saw. **Steve Garlock** and **Frank Pandora, Esq.,** are two of the best strategists and partners I ever met. Together, along with Board Chairman **Gerry Mayo,** the great and wonderful **Dr. Nick Baird** (now Director of the Department of Health for the State of Ohio) and Chief Financial Officer **Bill Wilkins**, we developed the entire U.S.Health system (now renamed OhioHealth) from a single hospital organization to the successful and complex multi-hospital system it is today. It was there that the seeds of the Healing Hospital were planted and developed. It was also there that I met,

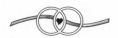

and here would like to acknowledge the guidance of, the late, great **Rev. Bob Davis.** His compassionate contributions to the work of healing care in hospitals and in communities are acts of kindness that continue to send ripples of love throughout the country.

When the New Healing Hospital was launched in early 2001, there was a good chance it would have failed immediately without the skillful and creative support provided by **Debby Koch,** former Senior Vice President at Baptist. She was trying to live the New Healing Hospital long before I arrived. Her efforts helped to spread the concept through the hospital and into the community. Her charm, her spirit, and her leadership continue to ensure that the concept and its expression are lived out each day. The banners she designed still hang from lampposts surrounding Baptist Hospital. They proclaim, "Discover the New Healing Hospital." I hope that you will do exactly that in the pages of this book — and that you will seek to promote the work of loving care wherever you live and work.

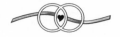

ENDNOTES

1 Henri Nouwen, *Reaching Out* (New York: Doubleday, 1975), p. 66.

2 Ibid., p. 67.

3 Dr. Rollo May, *Love and Will* (New York: Bantam Doubleday, 1969).

4 "In the Line of Duty: The FBI Murders" (NBC, 1988).

5 Nouwen, *Reaching Out,* p. 65.

6 Luke 10:25-37, Matthew 22:34-40, Mark 12:28-34 (NRSV).

7 *Star Wars: Episode VI — Return of the Jedi* (Lucasfilm,1983), produced by George Lucas.

8 Rollo May, *Psychology and the Human Dilemma* (New York: Bantam Doubleday, 1967), p. 30.

9 Richard Glenn, Ph.D., *Transform, Twelve Tools for Life* (Nashville: Providence House Publishers, 2003).

10 *Wall Street Journal,* March 28, 2003; Dr. Relman is also the former editor of *The New England Journal of Medicine.*

11 Dr. James Canton, healthcare futurist. Excerpt from his speech to healthcare leaders at the International Picker Institute Seminar discussing the Human Genome project: "The Future of Healthcare in a High Tech World," July 16, 2003, Boston.

12 Nouwen, *Reaching Out,* p. 65.

13 *Susan and God* (1940), MGM, starring Joan Crawford, Nigel Bruce and Rita Hayworth, produced by Hunt Stromberg and directed by George Cukor.

14 *U.S. News & World Report,* August 4, 2003.

15 Canton, "The Future of Healthcare..."

16 American Hospital Association Statistics for 2001.

17 CDC National Center for Health Statistics (2000).

18 J.D. Salinger, *Catcher in the Rye* (New York: Random House, 1945, 1951), p. 277.

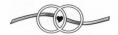

19 Nancy Moore and Henrietta Komras, *Patient-Focused Healing: Integrating Caring and Curing in Health Care* (San Francisco: Jossey-Bass Publishers, 1993), p. 53.

20 Speech to the National Research Council/Picker, Boston, July, 2002.

21 American Medical Association Principles of Ethics, June 2001, Principle 1.

22 Rollo May, *Psychology and the Human Dilemma* (New York: Bantam Doubleday, 1967), p. 31.

23 The well-known story *The Sorcerer's Apprentice* was written in 1897 by Paul Dukas (1865-1935), who was in turn inspired by a poem of the same name written by Johann Goethe in 1779. The story was further popularized by Walt Disney through his great feature-length cartoon *Fantasia*.

24 Parker J. Palmer, *Let Your Life Speak: Listening for the Voice of Vocation* (San Francisco: Jossey Bass, 2000), p. 62.

25 From the film *A Servant's Heart*, produced and directed by Erie Chapman and filmed under the direction of Van Grafton (Baptist Healing Hospital Trust, 2001).

26 Sallie McFague, *Life Abundant* (Minneapolis: Fortress Press, 2001), p. 202.

27 Quoted in *Modern Healthcare*, June 23, 2003, p. 76.

28 Robert Frost, "Two Tramps in Mud Time" (last stanza).

29 David Whyte, *The Heart Aroused: Poetry and the Preservation of the Soul in Corporate America* (New York: Currency Doubleday, 1994), p. 298.

30 McFague, *Life Abundant*, pp. 12, 20.

31 Black Elk, *Black Elk Speaks,* as told through John Neihardt (Lincoln: University of Nebraska Press, 1961), p. 43.

32 Czeslaw Milosz, *New and Collected Poems* 1931-2001 (New York: HarperCollins Publishers, 2001).

33 See Aaron Beck, M.D., et al., *Cognitive Therapy of Depression* (New York: The Guilford Press, 1987).

34 Moore and Komas, *Patient-Focused Healing*, p. 195.

35 I am indebted to my associate, David Cox, for bringing Gadamer's work to my attention.

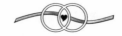

36 Hebrews 13:2 (NRSV).

37 Daniel E. Moerman, Ph.D., and Wayne B. Jones, M.D., "Deconstructing the Placebo Effect and Finding the Meaning Response," *Annals of Internal Medicine* 136, no. 6 (19 March 2002): 471-476.

38 Ibid., p. 473.

39 Ibid.

40 Rainer Maria Rilke, *Book of Hours: Love Poems to God* (New York: Riverhead Books, 1997).

41 Howard L. Harrod, "An Essay on Desire," *Journal of the American Medical Association,* 289, no. 7 (February 12, 2003): 813.

42 Nouwen, *Reaching Out,* p. 61.

43 Simone Weil, *Waiting for God* (New York: Perennial/Harper Collins Publishers, 2000).

44 Based on my estimates and best recollections but believed to be essentially correct.

45 Nelson Mandela — from his inauguration speech as President of South Africa.

46 Nouwen, *Reaching Out,* p. 64.

47 Steffie Woolhandler, M.D. M.P.H., et al, "Proposal of the Physicians' Working Group for Single-Payer National Health Insurance" (JAMA 2003; 290:798-805).

48 Nouwen, *Reaching Out,* p. 65.

49 Samuel Langhorne Clemens, *Adventures of Huckleberry Finn* (San Francisco: Chandler Publishing Company, 1885/1962), p. 148.

50 *Still Breathing* (Paramount, 1998).

51 Matthew 5-7 (NRSV).

52 The mission statement of the Baptist Healing Hospital Trust parallels this mission statement: **We are a caring ministry devoted to healing with love in the Christian tradition.**

53 All the data regarding Riverside and OhioHealth is based on my estimates and recollections.

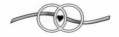

54 Based on estimates and best recollection.

55 This is according to secondhand reports that I have received.

56 Several sources reference this study, including the Milgram website at www.stanleymilgram.com

57 See an extensive report of this study at www.prisonexp.org

58 A good review of this work appears at www.geocities.com

59 *Sacred Work,* produced by Erie Chapman; filmed and co-edited by Van Grafton. Nashville: Baptist Healing Hospital Trust, 2001.

60 *Here Come the Girls* (1957).

61 Rollo May, *Love and Will* (Fountain Books, 1977).

62 See Appendix A for two pages of summary material on Care Partners and Scripting prepared by the Health Care Advisory Board, Washington, D.C.

63 David Whyte, *Crossing the Unknown Sea — Work as a Pilgrimage of Identity* (New York: Riverhead Books, 2001), p. 54.

64 Nouwen, *Reaching Out,* p. 95.

65 Ibid.

66 From a Kennedy Press conference (July 17, 1963).

67 Whyte, *Crossing the Unknown Sea,* p. 54.

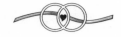

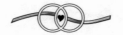

Study Guide

QUESTIONS

Part One — Love and the Higher Standard of the Healing Hospital

Chapter 1 — Opening Challenge
- How does the story of the housekeeper and the old man lay the foundation for a Healing Hospital?
- What is Radical Loving Care?
- How would you describe what a Healing Hospital is and what is accomplished by its creation?
- What are the three key symbols of a Healing Hospital and what do they signify?
- What kinds of results can be expected by establishing a Healing Hospital?
- What three prerequisites must be in place to establish a Healing Hospital?
- What is the significance of the story of the muder at Riverside in the context of Radical Loving Care?
- How does leadership handle emergencies in a Healing Hospital differently from a traditional hospital?
- What leadership styles do you see in this story?
- List Sacred Encounters in this story.

Chapter 2 — The Golden Thread
- What is the Golden Thread and why is the concept critical in a Healing Hospital?
- What are the differences between Robots and Humans, between Houses and Homes, and between Ordinary Hospitals and Healing Hospitals?

Chapter 3 — Five Challenges to a Healing Hospital
- Why do we need to educate hearts as well as minds?
- What are the five challenges to a Healing Hospital and how are they significant?
- What does it mean to deal with these challenges in balance?

Chapter 4 — Sacred Encounters, Sacred Work
"I Have Bad News"
- In what way were the three patterns of interaction by Dr. Krueger Sacred Encounters?
- What is the difference between the encounters she describes and more typical encounters between doctors and patients?
- What does this story tell us you about the life of hospital-based caregivers?

The Nurse and the Very Tiny Baby
- What does this story tell us about Sacred Encounters?
- What is the nature of unconditional love and what distinguishes it from other expressions of love?

Lois Powers' Power
- In what way were Lois Powers' encounters sacred?
- How was Lois able to bring passion to her work?
- How did she define her job?

Chapter 5 — The Servant's Heart
- What is the concept of the Servant's Heart and how does it help in the creation of a Healing Hospital?
- What is the relevance of the story of the Good Samaritan?
- How can an understanding of Glenn's "mental models" help transform our behavior toward others in a caregiving context?

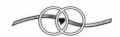

Chapter 6 — The Caring Community
- What does Dr. Hagan mean when he says we must transform our hospitals into "caring communities"?
- How can Care Circles and Care Partners shift culture?

Chapter 7 — The Layers of Meaning in Radical Loving Care
- What are the two layers of meaning that need to be understood in order to develop the continuous chain of light in Radical Loving Care?
- What is the importance of the German words Meinung and Bedeutung in the understanding of loving service?
- Why is the phrase Meaning Effect better than the phrase Placebo Effect in understanding the impact of loving care in a Healing Hospital?
- What is the Healing Formula and why is it important to understand Healing Care as a higher standard of care?
- What are liminal states and how does an understanding of them help us rethink our mental models about caregiving?

Chapter 8 — Presence and Affirmation
- Why is presence so critical to all three core concepts in a Healing Hospital?
- How do presence and affirmation help build the continuous chain of light that is Radical Loving Care?
- What is the significance of Tracy and Michelle's Presence and Affirmation magic?

Chapter 9 — The Not-So-Surprising Outcomes of the Healing Hospital
- What is the difference between doing something because it is right and doing something because it achieves better outcomes?
- What are the kinds of outcomes that are experienced by the Healing Hospital approach?

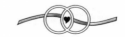

Part Two — The Blueprint for a Healing Hospital

Chapter 1 — Laying the Foundation
- What leadership commitment is required to lay the right foundation?
- What is the best way to secure board commitment to this work?
- How and when should the medical staff be engaged?
- What resource commitment is needed?
- How does a Healing Hospital foster good staffing practices?

Chapter 2 — Illuminating the Golden Thread of Healing
- What is missing in the ingredients for success at the large prestigious hospital referenced in the story?
- What is the great unfinished business of healthcare?
- How would behavior change in business meetings in a Healing Hospital?
- How do values like the Golden Thread help leaders impact the quality of clinical care as well as effective stewardship of financial resources?
- How can a vision be created that will galvanize the organization? What are the methods?
- What is the importance of the Southwest Airlines example and what is accomplished by the use of the "Rings of Care" model?
- How does it help to use images like "the dock, the boat, and in between?"
- How does the Frost poem enhance appreciation of this work?

Chapter 3 — Cultivating a Culture of Sacred Work
- What is Wave Theory and how does it help in understanding culture shift?
- What is the significance, here, of the first-day-of-school phenomenon?
- What caused the rise and fall at Riverside and what things does this teach us about building a Healing Hospital that will endure?
- What is the importance of dialogue, inquiry, and piloting, and what are the methods of implementing these approaches?
- What is Ripple Power and how can it be employed to affirm employee partners?

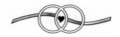

Chapter 4 — the Sacred Encounter in Practice
- How does the Encounter Window help our understanding of the practicality of Sacred Encounters?
- What brings about the Highest Level of Sacred Encounters?
- What are the kinds of Sacred Encounters that can be lived out in your work?
- How will you change your thinking in order to accomplish more Sacred Encounters?
- How will you help and affirm your staff in accomplishing these encounters?
- What is Magi Training and how does it support High Purpose Leadership?
- What are the Seven Practices of High Purpose Leadership and how can they be employed to advance the Healing Hospital?

Chapter 6 — Care Partners, Care Circles, and Integrative Medicine
- What are Care Partners and why are they important in advancing loving care?
- What are Care Circles? How can they be employed in regular work settings? How important are they to accomplishing change?
- What is the role of Integrative Medicine in healing patients and why is it important in a Healing Hospital?
- How can Presence training be implemented?

Chapter 7 — Sustaining the Servant's Heart
- What are the four steps to "filling the hospital with Servant's Hearts"?
- How does this concept affect productivity, turnover, union organizing, and employee morale?
- What is the Firelight Window and how can it be used to accomplish the four steps?
- What role do Humor and Play take in a Healing Hospital?

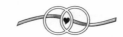

Conclusion

- What will it take to establish a Healing Hospital, or Healing Hospital approaches, in your work?
- How important could this be for patients?
- How are you going to carry this work forward?
- Personal Commitment
- Impact on Staff
- Impact on Leadership

APPENDIX A

Care Partner^{SM} Job Description

Position Summary

Works with the elderly patient and patient's family, facilitating needs and compassionately guiding them through their hospital experience. If system or process issues are encountered, Care Partner works toward solutions with other members of the health care team.

Education

College degree or equivalent.

Experience

- Demonstrated ability to read with comprehension, communicate verbally and in writing, and calculate simple mathematical problems.
- Prior hospital, assisted living, nursing home, and home health experience preferred, but not required.
- Personality and demeanor to deal with the public and assist ill, older, or distraught patients.

Skills

- Ability to read and comprehend (English) simple instructions and short correspondence.
- Interpersonal skills to care for patients in the elderly age group, on a continual basis.
- Excellent language and communication skills, both written and verbal.
- Basic knowledge of gerontology and special needs of patients.
- Proficiency in basic medical terminology.
- Guest relations, customer service, and interpersonal skills required.

Licensure

None required.

Essential Functions

- Assists in problem solving, medication administration, and acts as a sounding board with patient and hospital.
- Provides support and conflict resolution.
- Assists in maintaining safety needs of patient.
- Works with all members of the health care team and promotes a relationship of mutual respect.
- Demonstrates dignity with kindness and compassion to all patients, families, visitors and hospital staff.
- Demonstrates knowledge and skills in utilizing universal precautions and infection control policies.
- Demonstrates knowledge and skills regarding age appropriate care.
- Assists in maintaining physical and environmental comfort of the patient at all times.
- Facilitates trust and promotes understanding through careful listening and candid feedback.
- Responds promptly and appropriately in emergency situations.
- Provides a safe, comfortable environment for patients, families, and other staff members.

Working Conditions

Occasional exposure to one or more very unpleasant physical work conditions. Occasional exposure to serious injury. Regular and routine exposure to occupational hazards or contagious disease that require special precautions, including exposure to blood and body fluids that require precautions taken through most of working day.

Physical Effort

Occasionally requires light physical effort as in continuous standing or repeated changes of positions within the work routine.

Source: Baptist Hospital, Nashville, Tenn.; Health Care Advisory Board interviews.

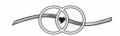

Care Partner^{SM} Scripting Guide

Presurgical Phone Call	
• Introduce Care Partner Program • Reassure patient • Arrange to meet patient before procedure	• "I'm _____, your continuous Care Partner across your stay at the hospital. All of our patients over 65 receive a Care Partner to discuss concerns, answer questions, or just to provide a little extra support." • "The hospital is a big place, and you'll see a lot of faces. It's my goal to make it feel like a much smaller place." • "Who's conducting the procedure? Oh yes, I've known Doctor _____ for years; you are in excellent hands." • "What time are you coming in?...Ok, after you arrive, they'll take you to the Welcome Center, then on to the admissions area where I'll meet you. I'll see you in the admissions area around 7 a.m." • "Are any family members coming with you?" • "Do you know about our valet parking service?" • "Do you have any questions? Is there anything on your mind?"

Presurgical Meeting in Admissions Area	
• Introduce Care Partner to patient and family • Explain process, from presurgery through recovery. • Discuss recovery, addressing patient and family concerns • Set expectations for recovery	• "Hi, I'm _____. We spoke on the phone yesterday; I'll be your care partner across your stay." • "How are you feeling this morning?" • "You be sure to concentrate on healing, I'll take care of your family and keep them informed." • "I'll see you when you return from surgery."

Conversations with Family in Waiting Area During Surgery	
• Reassure family members • Warn patients that constant overhead pages should not concern them • Provide contact number for any questions or concerns • Speak to OR staff if family has not received any updates	• "Have you received any updates from the nurses yet? Let me speak to a nurse and find out how the procedure is going." • "The procedure should be completed in the next hour." • "Don't be distracted by the pages you'll hear." • "Please call me at any time if you have any questions. Here is my card."

Post-Surgical Visits in Patient Room	
• Provide patient with 24-hour contact number • Encourage questions • Emphasize the importance of eating • Learn about normal eating habits to determine if food is being delivered at an appropriate time	• "How did you rest?" • "Is your pain medication working?" • "How did your family sleep?" (If they stayed at the hospital) • "Do you have any questions or concerns? Is there anything on your mind?" • "Are you happy with the food choices?" • "Would you like a drink/popsicle?" • "Is there anything else I can do for you? I have the time." • "Please call me at any time if there's anything I can do. Here is my card."

Source: Baptist Hospital, Nashville, Tenn.; Health Care Advisory Board interviews.

(Prepared by the Health Care Advisory Board Based on information provided by Baptist Hospital, Nashville, Tennessee)

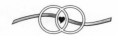

APPENDIX B

Key Slides:

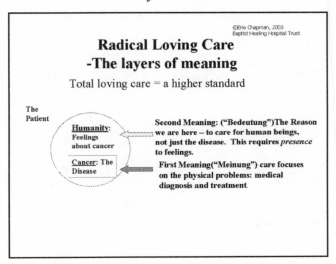

Radical Loving Care
-The layers of meaning

Total loving care = a higher standard

The Patient

Humanity: Feelings about cancer

Cancer: The Disease

Second Meaning: ("Bedeutung")The Reason we are here – to care for human beings, not just the disease. This requires *presence* **to feelings.**

First Meaning("Meinung") care focuses on the physical problems: medical diagnosis and treatment.

The Golden Thread
— *History & Tradition*

- **History is both a building block and a tool to teach.**

- **The golden thread of healing tradition is loving care.**

- **Our traditions inform us of who we should be and they press upon us the questions: "Are we who we say we are?" "How can we become who we seek to be?"**

- **We need to illuminate our shared tradition of loving care.**

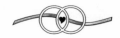

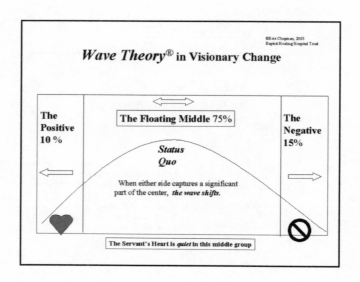

The Care Circles slide:

Care Circles

©Eric Chapman, 2003
Baptist Healing Hospital Trust

- Care circles are made up of 10-12 partners who meet regularly (weekly or monthly) to:
  - Check in with each other on personal and work life
  - Discuss the practice of particular tools that advance healing care.
- Consider impact of language
- Consider impact of leader's role in "setting the agenda" and determining focus

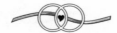

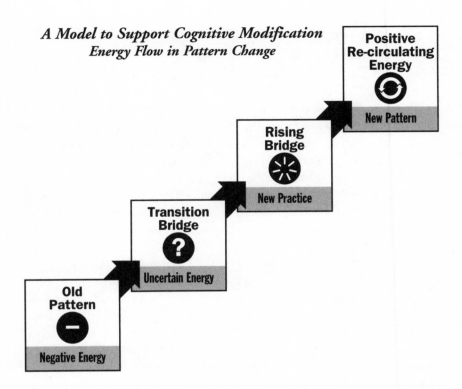

A Model to Support Cognitive Modification
Energy Flow in Pattern Change

Example — Monday Mornings: I experience negative energy every seven days on Monday mornings. To change this, I first need to become aware of the fact that I am generating the negative energy with my own thought pattern and that this can be changed if I establish a new thought pattern around Mondays. In the transition period, I may try out new ways of thinking about Mondays, but my energy may remain uncertain and I may give up if I don't find a good alternative easily. If I cross the bridge successfully and enter a new practice, I will feel a sense of rising energy. But the new pattern is not yet ingrained. After a period of effort, however, the new pattern takes hold and positive energy recirculates. Monday mornings have now become a positive experience and this positive feeling will regenerate on its own.

This model applies in a work context in renaming all the negative pictures around hospital work. Therefore, strangers in patient gowns become my suffering brothers and sisters and work becomes sacred.

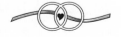

A BRIEF HISTORY OF
THE NEW HEALING HOSPITAL
AND THE BAPTIST HEALING HOSPITAL TRUST

In early 2001, **Erie Chapman**, then President of Baptist Hospital System, formally announced the concept for what he called a New Healing Hospital at a leadership meeting of over a hundred managers. The ideas that make up this concept had been in the formative stages for many years. Many hospitals have mission statements and plans that sound like a Healing Hospital. The true difference comes in the degree to which these plans are lived out. The Healing Hospital concept is about living out what we truly believe about loving service to patients and loving relationships among staff members.

The leadership team that developed the Healing Hospital concept and guided Baptist during the period of the late 1990s through the end of 2001 included several key players starting with Mr. Chapman; **Jeff Kaplan**, Executive Vice President; **Paul Moore**, Chief Operating Officer; **Tracy Wimberly**, Chief Mission Officer; **Debby Koch**, Senior Vice President, **Susan Crutchfield**, Senior Vice President; **James O'Keefe**, Chief Financial Officer; and **Stephanie Zembar**, Chief Legal Counsel. **Gayle Malone,** Esq., also provided key support. An intensive effort was focused on the successful turnaround that took place during this time.

It is important to note something very few people ever fully understood at the time — and that was how close Baptist Hospital came to declaring bankruptcy and going out of business. The ending months of 1998 were a dark time for Baptist Hospital since a loss of $73 million dollars for FY '98 had been reported in early October. The president of the hospital, Mr. Chapman, called other possible health system buyers to see if they might bail out the system by buying it. He got a flat turndown from every buyer he called. Not a single system was willing to pay a single dime for Baptist. It was then that the hospital system and Baptist Hospital in particular, a venerable Nashville institution employing over three thousand people, came the closest to closing.

After a dramatic recovery headlined by the Healing Hospital initiative, however, the system was subsequently sold for hundreds of millions of dollars at the end of 2001. This means that the value had gone from 0 to hundreds of millions in three years! In essence, the entire sale price and thus all of the assets of the Baptist Healing Hospital Trust, was created in a three-year period from 1998–2001, building on the base of a wonderful hospital

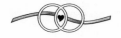

that had developed over more than eighty years! This kind of turnaround requires strength when times are the hardest and that is exactly what came from the entire Baptist Hospital organization.

An intensive effort was focused across several areas. First, as many non-patient-related assets as possible were sold or discarded. These included the sale of one of the System's five hospitals, Three Rivers, the sale of several pieces of real estate, and the return of nearly a hundred physician practices to their original physician owners.

Inside the hospital, a deep effort was instituted to restore and strengthen employee morale and to strengthen patient and physician satisfaction. The story of this work, including its foundation and direction, is told extensively in *Radical Loving Care.*

The sale also required the work of a talented negotiating team on behalf of Baptist. This team was lead by Jeff Kaplan and was also made up of board member **Scott Jenkins**, Jim O'Keefe, and Stephanie Zembar. This team did a brilliant job. Their successful negotiation led to a fair price for both sides and has led to ongoing good relations between the organizations.

It is important to remember the history of Baptist Hospital itself. The heritage of Baptist Hospital begins in 1918 when it was founded as **Protestant Hospital**. The hospital changed its name to Baptist in 1948 when that denomination took over responsibility for the Christian ministry of the organization. **Dr. James Sullivan** and **Mr. Jack Massey** were initial leaders of this effort. In an early meeting of the reformed organization, board member **A. Roy Greene** articulated the sense of mission these founders felt:

> *Mr. Greene stated that the transfer of the Hospital to Baptists presented us with an opportunity to reach the souls of men through the ministry of healing their bodies . . .*

Dr. Sullivan once said, "The most important things we do, we do unknowingly." He could not, of course, have specifically foreseen the impact of his own early work in the re-founding of Baptist Hospital — a legacy that lives on to this day through the work of caregivers.

The Baptist Healing Hospital Trust was created at the end of 2001 as the sale of the hospital became imminent and there was a need to determine a use for the proceeds of the sale. The assets of Baptist Hospital System are a community resource. The reason most of the income from the Baptist Healing Hospital Trust is dedicated to loving care in hospitals is

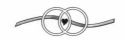

that the money came from exactly that source.

The biggest increase in the value of the Baptist Hospital System happened between late 1998 and 2001. This is the time during which leadership was fully engaged in carrying out the mission of loving service to staff and patients. That mission had been somewhat obscured during the mid-1990s when many resources were focused away from direct patient care. As the original mission of the organization was restored, the value of the organization began to climb.

Still, the Board of Trust, under the outstanding leadership of Chair **Virgil Moore**, wisely understood that after the hospital returned to break-even, it was still in very fragile economic shape. It was time to sell — and sell to an organization that had the fiscal stability to sustain both the economic strength of the system and its Christian mission of loving service. The buyer turned out to be the Ascension Health System and Saint Thomas Health Services. Their Christian mission is both strong and long, and the board believed they would be the best choice to carry forward the ministry of the Baptist Hospital System.

It was **Willie Davis**, former Treasurer of the Board of Trust, who first suggested a particular kind of formula to help ensure the continuation of the Baptist Healing Hospital mission. Virgil Moore, Chairman, along with Vice Chairman **Ken Ross,** Secretary **Ed Moody,** and **Dr. Robert Norman**, insisted on the continuation of the Baptist name, and **Dr. Keith Hagan** provided invaluable physician leadership throughout this period. Mr. Davis's formula proposed that each year for seven years from the date of sale, 70% of the net income of the Trust (after expenses), be paid to Saint Thomas Health Services designated specifically for Baptist Hospital. This payment would be subject to two conditions. The first condition was that Saint Thomas had to maintain the name Baptist on the main campus at 2000 Church Street. The second condition is that the new owners of Baptist Hospital had to demonstrate to the satisfaction of the Trust board that the Healing Hospital mission was continued and advanced at Baptist.

During 2002, the first year of the Trust's full operation, the staff working with **Julie O'Connor**, mission officer for Saint Thomas at Baptist, performed an extensive review. Saint Thomas Health Services successfully fulfilled both conditions and received a grant of $1,288,000. The Trust looks forward to continuing this partnership with Saint Thomas Health Services throughout the balance of the obligated term. It is hoped that this seven-year period will provide for adequate time to plant the Healing Hospital deeply at Baptist so that it will endure beyond the period of the

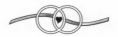

legal obligation.

The community owes a deep debt of gratitude to the volunteer board members who have served so unselfishly — many of them for dozens of years. **DeVaughn Woods**, the longest-serving board member, began his term on the Baptist Hospital System Board in 1957! The names of some of these dedicated men and women are referenced herein. Yet it is impossible to list the full extent of their contribution to Baptist Hospital and to the Baptist Healing Hospital Mission that so distinguishes Christian service in hospital settings.

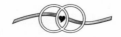

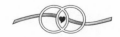

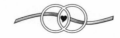

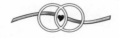

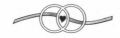

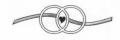